T0032200

HERBANA WITCH

A YEAR IN THE FOREST

Vivida

Vivida® trademark is the property of White Star s.r.l.
www.vividabooks.com

© 2023 White Star s.r.l.
Piazzale Luigi Cadorna, 6 - 20123 Milan, Italy
www.whitestar.it

This edition first published in 2023 by Red Wheel, an imprint of
Red Wheel/Weiser, LLC
With offices at
65 Parker Street, Suite 7
Newburyport, MA 01950
www.redwheelweiser.com

Graphic design and layout by
Due mani non bastano

Text by Cecilia Lattari
Illustrations by Alice Guidi
Translation by Alexa Ahernn of ICEIGeo, Milan

All rights reserved. No part of this publication may be reproduced or transmitted in any form or
by any means, electronic or mechanical, including photocopying, recording, or by any information
storage and retrieval system, without permission in writing from Red Wheel/Weiser, LLC.
Reviewers may quote brief passages.

Library of Congress Cataloging-in-Publication Data available upon request

ISBN 978-1-59003-539-9

Printed in China
1 2 3 4 5 6   25 24 23 22 21

This book contains advice and information for using herbs and other botanicals, and is not meant
to diagnose, treat, or prescribe. It should be used to supplement, not replace, the advice of your
physician or other trained healthcare practitioner. If you know or suspect you have a medical
condition, are experiencing physical symptoms, or if you feel unwell, seek your physician's
advice before embarking on any medical program or treatment. Readers are cautioned to follow
instructions carefully and accurately for the best effect. Readers using the information in this book
do so entirely at their own risk, and the author and publisher accept no liability if adverse effects
are caused.

HERBANA WITCH

WITCH

A YEAR IN THE FOREST

Cecilia Lattari

Illustrations by Alice Guidi

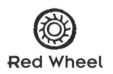

Red Wheel

H

18 Winter

52 Spring

ERBANA

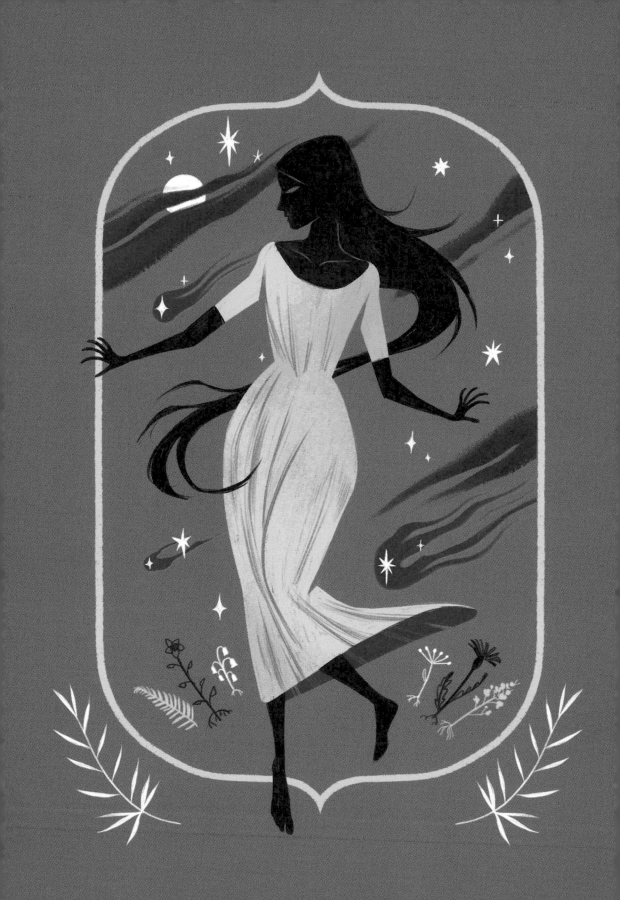

Ever since I was a girl,
I have heard the calling of herbs.
I remember playing with clover
and dandelion flowers that grew near
the house. I would rub them
on the garden wall around the house
to draw meadows and skies, flowers
and secret writings. I have always felt magic
is something natural, a flow that has led me,
over the years, to the practice
and study of herbs, to pay attention
to the language of animals and to be
enchanted, every year, by the changing
of seasons, their colors and gifts.
I am an herbana, without a doubt.
**But what does it mean
to be an herbana witch?**

WHO IS THE HERBANA WITCH?

IN ITALIAN, THE WORD STREGA MEANS WITCH. THE LATIN AND GREEK WORDS STRIGA AND STRIX, RESPECTIVELY, MEAN "OWL, A NOCTURNAL ANIMAL." THIS ANIMAL WAS ASSOCIATED WITH ATHENA, THE GODDESS OF WISDOM, AND THUS INDICATES THAT A WITCH IS A WISE FIGURE WHO KNOWS HOW TO ACT IN HARMONY WITH THE FORCES OF NATURE.

THE HERBANA WITCH knows the language of nature and cyclical time. She knows how to use nature and its expression to help bring harmony and healing to living beings. Others may see her as an herbalist or as an expert in gardens and horticulture. The herbana witch possesses those skills, but her defining quality is her profound relationship with nature. The herbana witch listens to nature's messages, understands its symbolism, and is aware of the healing and nourishing properties of plants, flowers, and trees. She is an earth witch, just as the wise women of the past were.

She often knows folk enchantments, passed down by oral tradition and linked to the land. She probably lives on the outskirts of a city, in the countryside or near the woods. She follows the natural rhythm of the seasons and celebrates cyclical time.

The herbana witch is the goddess of small things. She can appreciate their sacredness, respects them, and knows how to find them. Her tools come from nature, like wands made of hazelnut or elder trees. She keeps jars full of harvested and dried herbs in an ever-plentiful pantry, including coffee beans ready to be ground and sunflower seeds for bread dough in the spring. Her magic is linked to her experience; it is not ceremonial or ritualistic. Her roots are in the practice of "signatures," a practice dating back to the time of Paracelsus. What is signatures? It is the art of knowing how to observe the signs and symbols found in the natural world and connecting them to humans, to find healing relationships, restore balance and heal. One example is *Hypericum perforatum*, or the St. John's Wort plant, due to its leaves, which when observed against the light are perforated; therefore, it was associated with wounds and the plant's ability to heal them. Modern medicine has shown us that this is the case, and like in this example, many references reveal the macrocosm in the microcosm, confirming the ancient wisdom of Hermes Trismegistus: "As above, so below."

The herbana witch knows the best time to plant and transplant seeds is with the waxing moon, never the waning moon. She feels this instinctively, or she has learned it through experience. She can recognize the footsteps of the fox and the voice of the boar. She can talk to cats and plants. She lives mindfully, aware that humans are not the only inhabitants of Earth. The herbana witch is familiar with both the visible and invisible worlds. She loves to make ointments, balms, and lotions. Her herbal teas taste of the forest and the moon. She does not live far from you. If you are reading this book, perhaps you too hear the herbs speaking. It is time to listen carefully.

In this book, you will follow the life and practices of an herbana witch who lives near the woods. You will discover the key plants of each season, sacred animals, a few secret recipes, and practices and activities for different moments in time, completing a full cycle of a year. There's only one thing to know before reading: magic is all around us. We just have to learn to recognize it.

FOLLOW THE PATH OF THE HERBS

TO BE AN HERBANA WITCH MEANS CHOOSING TO FOLLOW THE PATH OF THE HERBS. THIS PATH IS VERY SIMILAR TO THE LITTLE TRAIL THAT LED INTO THE WOODS FROM YOUR CHILDHOOD MEMORIES. PERHAPS IT WAS A DIRT ROAD DOTTED WITH CHAMOMILE AND VERBENA THAT MEANDERED THROUGH THE BRUSH BELOW THE GARDEN.

LIKE THE HERBANA WITCH, perhaps when you were young you, too, would rub flowering wild mint between your fingers as you took the path so that the scent would linger with you on your walk, like some kind of talisman. This path might have been by the sea, enveloped by the licorice-scented helichrysum; or maybe it was your wild herb path in the city through that space called the "third landscape," the area where wild and cultivated meet.

Herb trails appear in big cities, too. They are marked by delicate, unruly poppies, sun-yellow dandelions, or the lunar and mysterious mugwort that grows near an abandoned railroad track, inside an uninhabited house, beyond an open gate, or by a rusty old plaque. To follow an herb trail, you must first be able to see it. This is the first requirement.

Some people observe the herbs naturally, with respect and curiosity. Perhaps you too do not feel lonely when you have a plant near you. You may feel that the plant is alive and you can form a relationship with it as a living being. To go down this path, two other things are required: curiosity and a spirit of observation.

Try to look at each plant as if you do not know it, as if you have never seen it before. Even if you are familiar with its properties, try to do what our ancestors did and develop your skills of observation and intuition, making connections between signs and symbols and what you see. Then, learn to observe with curiosity, investigate in a participatory way, and stay in touch with the plant. Following the herb path means discovering that there is a real relationship between plants and humans. Not only will you be able to communicate with plants and act in harmony with them, but they will also be able to enter into a relationship with you.

This means that each plant has its own voice, and it communicates in its own way. You can sharpen your senses and listen, discovering the reciprocity of this kind of dialogue. It is important to study the plant in relation to its environment. Like us, a plant is a part of its environment and will be affected by it, being a full expression of it. The herb path is often a home or pathway for the *genus loci*, or the spirit of place. This spirt is the feeling that pervades you when you are in a special place, made up of everything you see, hear, smell, and touch as well as the invisible parts. Here, choosing the herb path means choosing to look even where there seems to be nothing, to listen to a voice made of wind and leaves, to be caressed by the stars or the sun. To feel that we are part of a whole that we can call home.

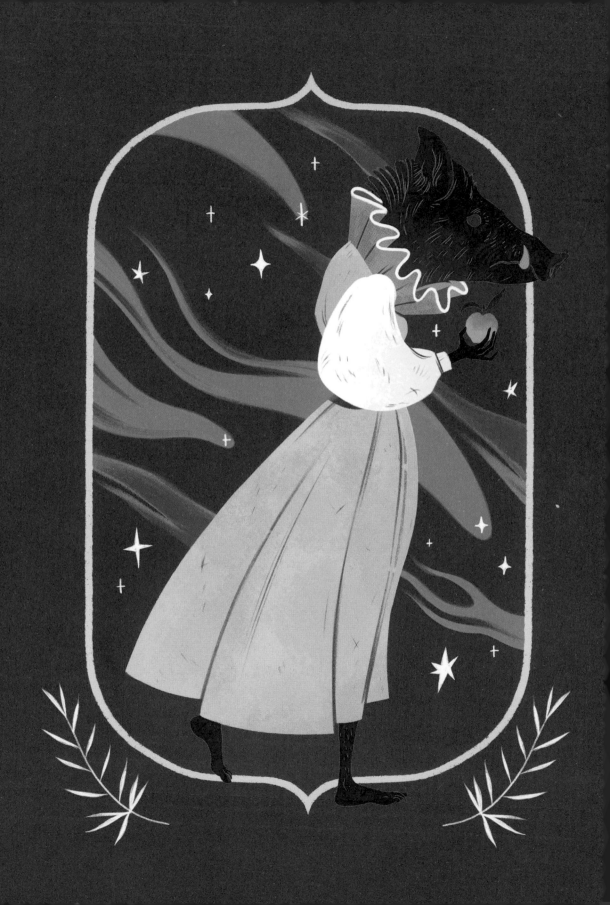

At dusk, on the border between
the herbana witch's garden
and the forest, a wild boar appears.
It is a female. She is not very big.
She hides among the last rays
of the sun and some fallen logs.
The herbana witch approaches;
only a metal net separates them.
She brings with her some apples,
some dry bread, and the too-ripe plums
that have fallen from the tree.
She lays them on the ground,
and the animal eats them,
looking at her with a mixture
of curiosity and awe. The herbana witch
kneels, stares straight into
the boar's eyes, and whispers to her,
**"Don't trust humans too much.
Stay wild."**

THE EDGE

SINCE THE EARLIEST OF TIMES, PLACES AT THE EDGE HAVE BEEN SPECIAL. THAT WHICH LIES BETWEEN THE VILLAGE AND THE FOREST IS NOT QUITE WILD BUT NOT QUITE ORDINARY EITHER. FAIRY TALES HAVE TOLD US OF THE WISE OLD WOMAN WHO LIVES ON THE EDGE OF THE WOODS. PERHAPS SHE IS SOME SORT OF HEALER OR HERBAL EXPERT.

ON THE EDGE lives the person who presides over rites of passage and uses ancient wisdom to heal. The edge is a space on the threshold, a place of possibility, where we can see things from a different perspective. It is the place where the real and the magical meet. It is an unruly space where weeds grow free and animals watch and protect those who live there. In ancient times, all rituals took place at the edge.

They marked the stages of life and celebrated the mutations of time or nature, and also marked the spaces and boundaries of the community. Here initiates learned the arts of life and experienced death and rebirth through the performance of these rituals.

Fairy tales, which are powerful tools for recounting life and connecting with the imaginary, came to life on the edge. And it is always where the mentor, the witch, the fairy, or the sorceress live. Where we find the ogre and the wolf. And where the shaman and herbana witch call home. She is outside the ordinary community, but she is as connected to it and the real world as she is to the hidden world.

She maintains privileged contact with ancestors, and often has power over the present and an ability to read subtle signs, to obtain clues and suggestions about the future. She knows nature and its forces and can heal using herbs and her knowledge. She is the one who administers rituals and guides transitions. When the edge is understood not only as a physical space but also as a condition for those who are different or marginalized, it becomes a place that should be inhabited with awareness, as bell hooks explained in many of her writings.

The edge is thus a space that stands in opposition to the tenets of the majority, to what is ordinary; it is at times a difficult space, but if it is experienced as a space of resistance and revolution, it is a space that is rich in potential, freedom, and possibility. Herbs are our masters in this as well. Weeds prefer the edge, where they can grow undisturbed, spreading their seeds to the wind.

Weeds teach us rebellion, which is not necessarily an act of destruction, but rather one of creation. Weeds add value to the ordinary because they succeed in preserving a different perspective, seeing the world and its resources from an alternative point of view. It is here, on the edge where the dream world and reality meet, that the power of the herbana witch and the wisdom of the shaman take root. Just think of the mist that envelops the forest, gradually creating a boundary between the visible and the invisible.

Persephone, the daughter of Demeter, is the goddess who inhabits the edge. She lives for part of the year on Earth, and for the remainder lives in the underworld. Just like the seed, she knows both worlds because she frequents the threshold that divides and unites them. That is why the herbana witch is not only an herbalist or healer, but also a mentor and a shaman, one who knows how to travel between worlds. To know and inhabit the edge is to experience closeness with something that may be different from us, and to learn from it.

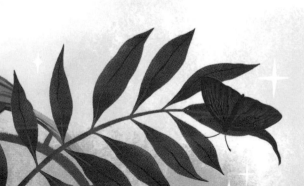

THE LAND AND TOOLS OF THE WITCH

THE HERBANA WITCH LIKES TO LIVE CLOSE TO NATURE. ONLY HERE CAN SHE HAVE DAILY CONTACT WITH PLANTS AND ANIMALS. THIS DOES NOT MEAN THAT EVERY HERBANA WITCH LIVES IN THE MIDDLE OF THE WOODS. WHEREVER SHE IS, SHE KNOWS HOW TO FIND A WAY TO CONNECT WITH NATURE.

QUITE OFTEN, witches can be found in the city. They love the "third landscape," places that contain wild plants, unexpected and domestic animals, and magical resources. The outdoor landscape is important because it tells us so much about the plants we may find and what animals and energy we will encounter. However, the land of the herbana witch does not only refer to external land, but also—and more importantly— the internal landscape. This inner landscape is made up of emotions, memories, and thoughts. We need to tap into these senses in order to get in touch with the herbs, to discover the path of magic that will lead us to them. The map that guides the herbana witch is sensory; we can activate our inner landscape by relying on all our senses. When our senses are activated, we learn about the plants we encounter and the places we inhabit. We discover new sounds and we catch glimpses of something we have never seen before even in the most well known places that we walk past every day.

To map the land as best she can, the herbana witch always carries a notebook with her in which she can record her observations, gathering times, how the light changes during the day, and how the forest changes during the seasons.

You can do as she does and start exploring your own land in new ways. Look for wild spaces, inspiration, and new stories in your everyday environment, and watch as the magic unfolds before you. The herbana witch has a few very simple tools, and she is rarely without them.

The first is a woven basket, which she uses to collect herbs, roots, flowers, and berries depending on the season; it is not very large, because she collects only what she needs, respecting the forest and its inhabitants.

Along with the basket, she has a pair of sharp, handy scissors, to cut the herbs without damaging them, so that they may finish their growing cycle.

The herbana witch always has a mortar. This is where she crushes and grinds herbs and resins to prepare incense and herbal teas. Her pantry has no shortage of glass jars, bottles, and vials where she stores healing balms, medicinal teas, and seeds for planting the following year. She has a small supply of beeswax which she uses to make her candles or to thicken ointments and salves; a cauldron or a large Dutch oven with a few vivid flowers painted on it, for simmering a warm, comforting soup; cookies, apples, and nuts for the wild animals; a silver bell, left at an oak branch, which rings for the fairy dance.

The herbana witch has watchful eyes, likes to be aloof but has many trusted friends, is a sensitive introvert and sometimes prefers the company of fireflies to that of humans. But if you knock on her door, there will always be a cup of tea waiting and someone willing to listen to your story. Of course, the herbana witch loves stories, and she spins them throughout the year—in the woods, as she listens to them in the tales of foxes and elves, the footsteps of wolves, and from Mother Mountain.

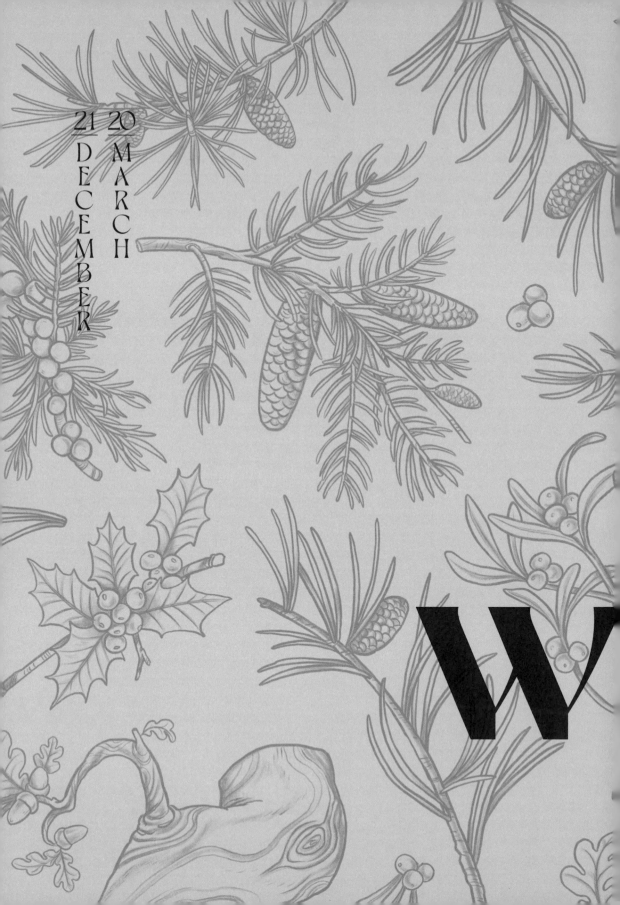

21 DECEMBER
20 MARCH

W

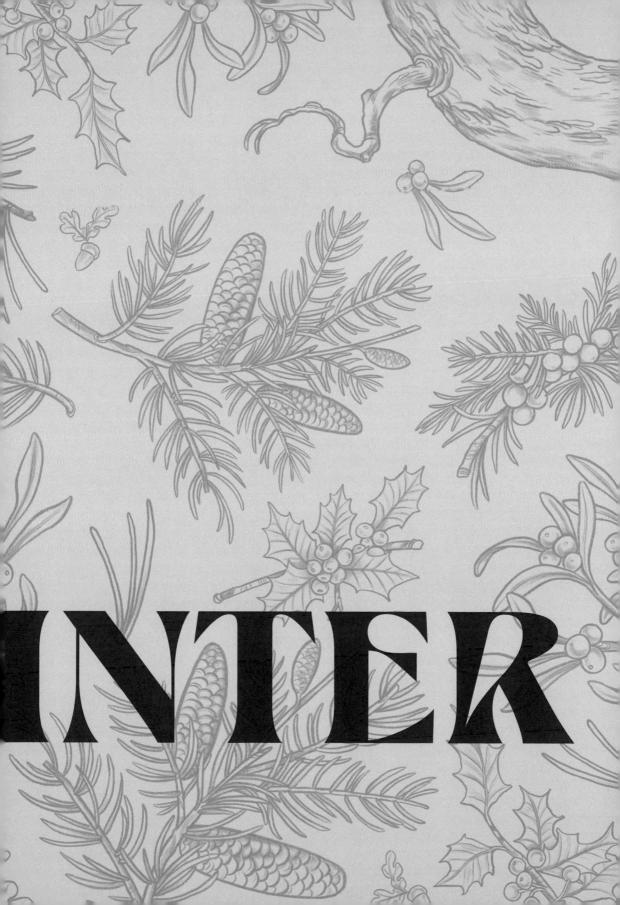

INTER

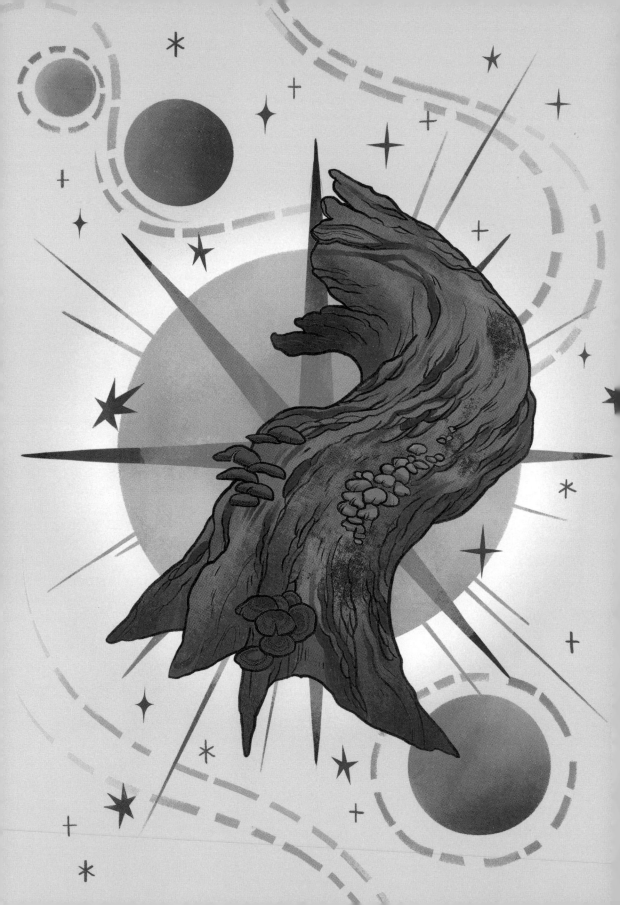

Winter invites protection and rest. Everything is silent in the woods.

The barks of trees stand out with their unique patterns that you run your fingers across during walks in the cold, clear air. The stems and trunks of plants can be herbaceous or woody, the latter meaning they are protected by bark, the outermost part of the plant. Bark is the covering of the trunk, branches, and root. On closer inspection, the bark is almost like a human's skin. It is the place where the exchange and contact between outside and inside takes place. Even in the winter, when everything is still, stories told before sleeping, dreams, plans, and wishes are exchanged. The herbana witch knows the dreams of plants and their alphabet of petals and seeds. The bark is protection, shelter, home. It is linked to the history of time, its furrows reminiscent of wrinkles, marks capable of telling the story of life.

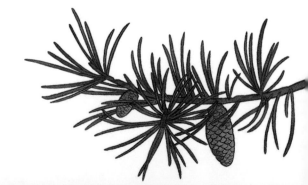

Snow in the forest emerges like a dream.

On a winter's night, the trees are bare; they have dropped their leaves in autumn and are now exposed, revealing the knots and patterns of their wood. Then, in the morning, when the herbana witch wakes up and looks out the window with a cup of strong black tea in her hands, everything is snowy. The sound of snow is a magical silence, interrupted at times by the wind. It creates new melodies in the branches, with the snow falling into small piles, a gentle beating from the heart of the forest. The beeches (*Fagus sylvatica*) and maples (*Acer*) are covered in a white cloak, as are the birches (*Betula alba*), whose very pale bark blends in with the snow. The evergreen firs (*Abies pectinata*) have weathered the night storm gracefully and now remain quiet and mysterious in the deep green of their needles. The holly (*Ilex aquifolium*) smiles on snowy mornings. The bright red of its berries is that of fairy tales, stories of fairy girls and the spindles for casting spells.

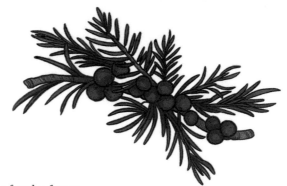

Winter is a quiet time for the forest, when seeds rest in the dark earth. It is a good time to plan, write, take notes and rest, as the herbana witch well knows. During this season the hearth fire continues to burn, the wood crackles in the stove, and the cinnamon-scented sugar cookies are ready for tea. During the winter, it is nice to learn something new, to study, to read that book that has been waiting for us for a long time. Learn a new art with your hands, such as embroidery, crocheting, or knitting, or carving a spoon from a piece of wood. With rest, you can slow down and carry out your daily activities quietly once you have returned to your nest. Winter, which is the most difficult season in the woods, reminds us of gratitude for all we have, for comfort and warmth.

The snowflakes form perfect crystals, not one identical to the other, highlighting beauty, even when things are hard. The wolf approaches the herbana witch's house more often. She catches a glimpse at night, a sharp silhouette cutting through the garden, passing beyond the woods, carrying solitude in his role as a guide. The herbana witch greets him in her thoughts, squinting her eyes, and he almost seems to turn for a moment before disappearing into the darkness.

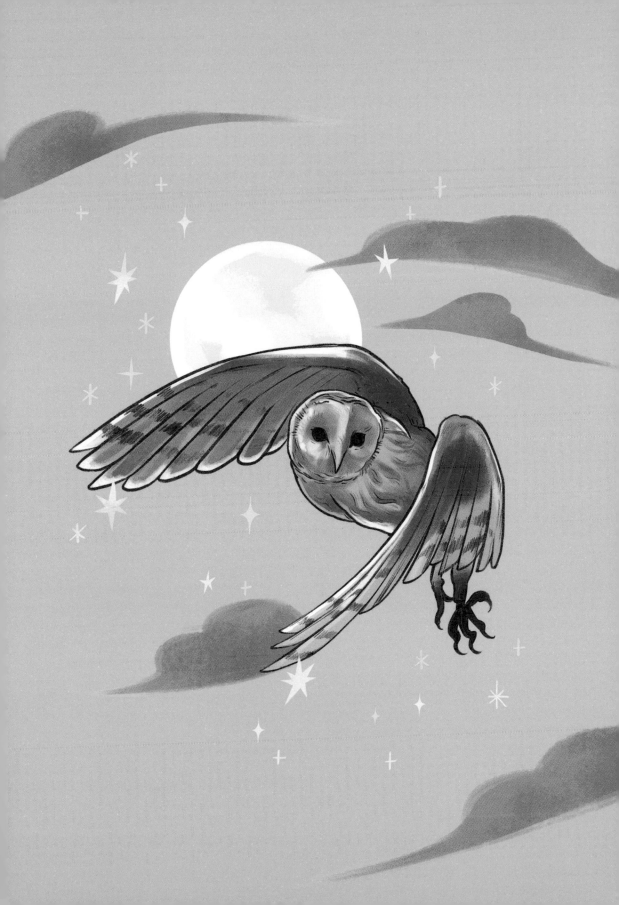

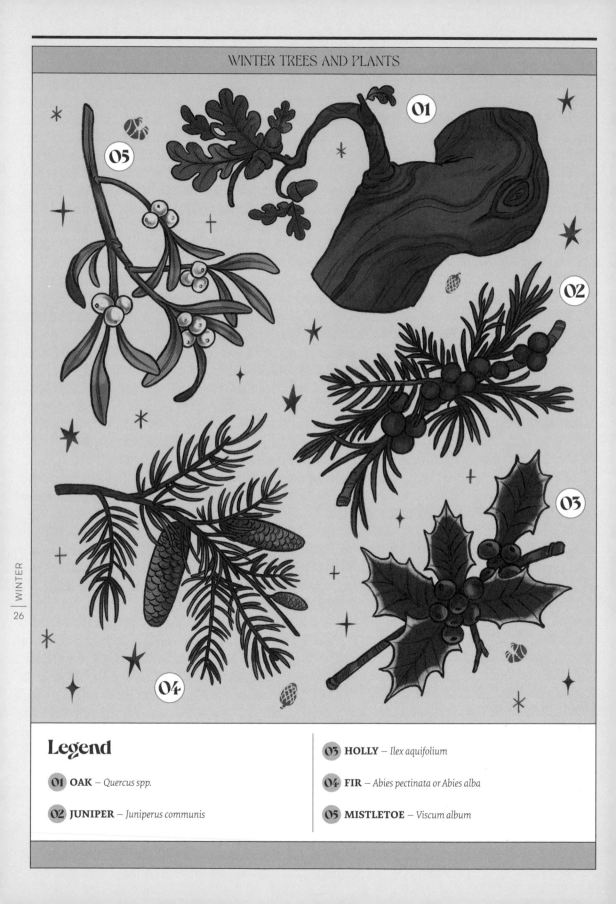

Legend

01 **OAK** – *Quercus spp.*

02 **JUNIPER** – *Juniperus communis*

03 **HOLLY** – *Ilex aquifolium*

04 **FIR** – *Abies pectinata or Abies alba*

05 **MISTLETOE** – *Viscum album*

Winter Trees and Plants

Winter plants are essential. Activity during this season is directed inward and underground, either in the root or in the seed waiting to sprout in spring. Winter plants are soothing and regenerative, and often have good effects on the bones. This season is closest to Saturn, which regulates life and presides over what is necessary, teaching the slowness and power of what will be born.

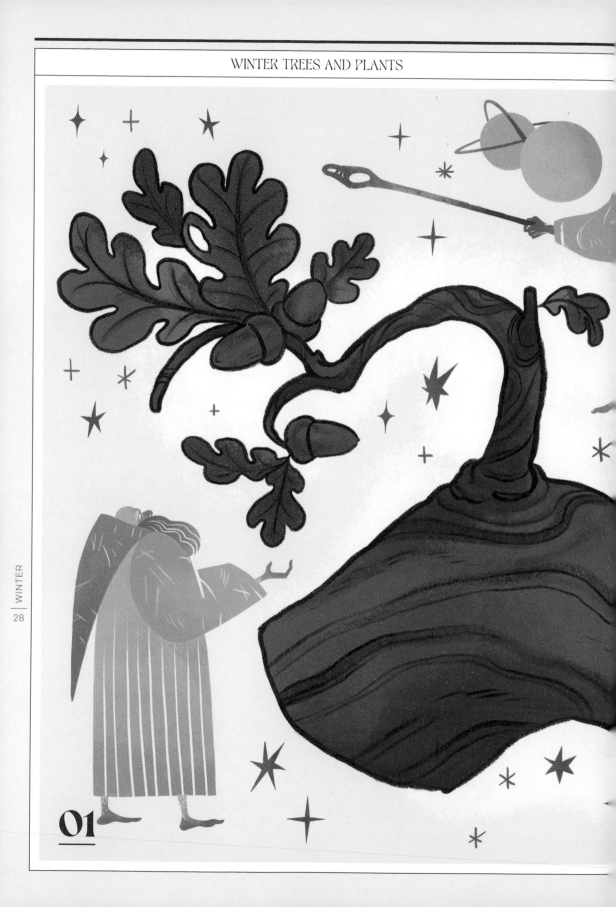

01

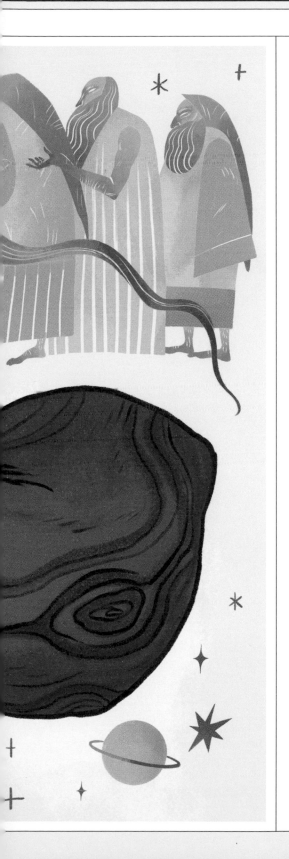

Oak

The oak, majestic and old, is a threshold tree between autumn and winter. The oak bark resembles the water in autumn, hollowed out by long furrows, in the shape of its curved acorns and in its leaves, sinuous and soft. But the oak is hard, woody, and impenetrable, bearing the mark of winter. It has slow growth and lives long. It exudes great wisdom and power. It is home and shelter to many animals: owls, squirrels, and dormice inhabit its mighty branches. It provides food for roe deer and wild boar, which feed on its acorns. It rarely lives in solitude; a community springs up around it. A symbol of strength and wisdom, a sacred tree for the Druids and very important to the Celts, it was also used for divination. People would read the movement of its leaves to receive advice and visions of the future. Tannin, a substance extracted from oak, is useful for treating eczema and frostbite. Tannin is also used to treat hides in tanning. A special flour is made from acorns. If roasted and prepared properly, acorns can also be used as a coffee substitute.

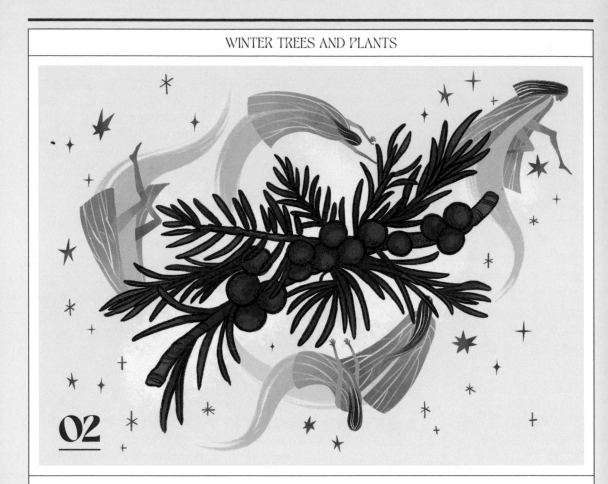

02

Juniper

Juniper is a pioneer plant. It grows and develops on new soil and prefers solitude. It has a winter disposition, which you can see in its leaves, which are needle-shaped and have a silver stripe down the center, reminiscent of snow and the harshness of the season. It has pointy leaves, which means picking the cones should be done with caution. The cones ripen in the fall and can be harvested year-round because they remain on the plant for a long time. In winter, they offer a unique flavor for seasonal dishes, from soups to roasts. The deep blue color of the cones represents depth and contemplation. Juniper has been associated since ancient times with the threshold, death, and contact with the Small Folk, or the fairy creatures that inhabit the forest. Juniper wood, which is very durable, was considered protective, and bundles of juniper were hung on the doors of houses to keep evil away. Juniper has antimicrobial, antiseptic, cleansing, and purifying properties. When added to food, it stimulates appetite and aids in digestion.

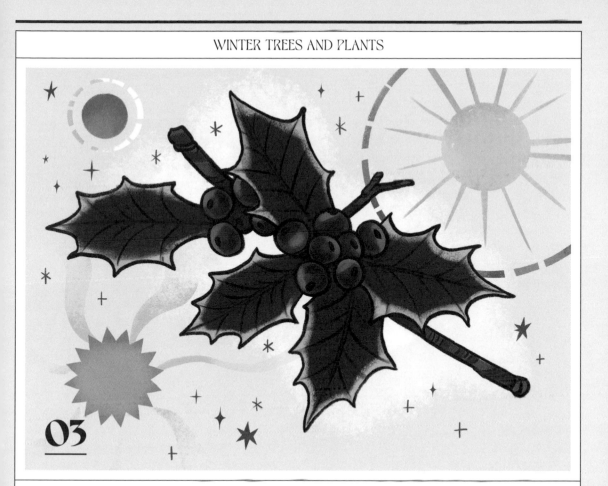

Holly

Holly belongs to the winter solstice. The ancient Romans wore amulets composed of this plant on the days leading up to the solstice, as it functions as a talisman. Holly is an evergreen, with glossy, leathery dark green leaves. The thorns on its leaves symbolize protection, whereas its red berries represent the sun returning after the longest nights of the year. Holly is very attached to the light. Its leaves bend when grown in shady areas, taking on a distinct curled appearance to better absorb the sun's rays. As the tree grows taller, reaching the sunlight more easily, the leaves stretch and spread. Holly is known as the "King of Winter." *The Holly King* of Celtic and British tradition presides over the darkest part of the year. Holly is one of Dr. Bach's remedies, as it allows for the transformation of anger into vital energy.

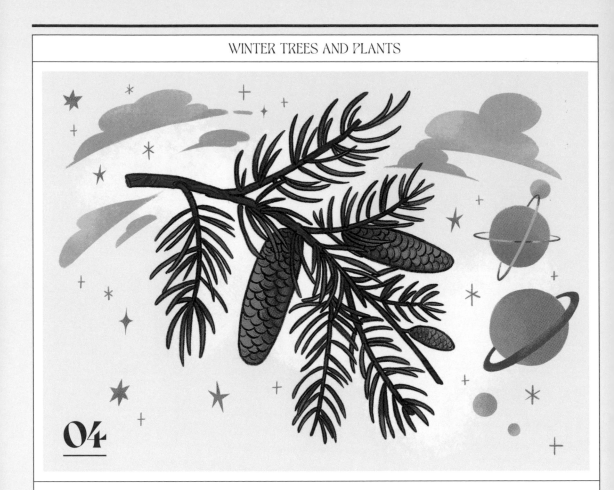

04

Fir

In Siberian mythology, the fir tree is the link between heaven and Earth. The shape of the tree, which stretches upwards, resembles an antenna. It is the plant that brings cosmic energy and messages to Earth. The fir is strong and graceful, capable of picking up subtle signs. It is a symbol of fertility because of the large number of pine cones it produces, and therefore, it was sacred to Artemis, goddess of the moon and forests, protector of births. The fir is very cold-hardy, growing at high altitudes. Like the holly, the fir is an evergreen. A symbol of the holiday season, it is brought into homes and adorned with lamps to mark the transition from darkness to light. It has soothing, expectorant properties and helps the respiratory tract in the case of colds. A fir tree has a strong, vital, saturnine skeleton-like structure. Since, as the saying goes, like is cured by like, fir bud-derivatives loosen joints and improve the skeletal system. Its shoots are rich in vitamin C and have a fresh, balsamic flavor.

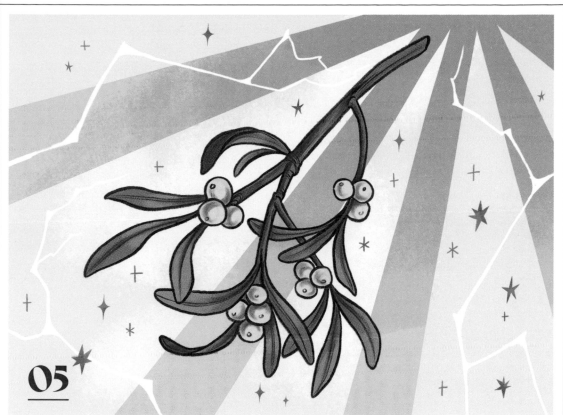

05

Mistletoe

Mistletoe is a peculiar plant. It appears in the dead of winter as a hanging shrub that seems to have no roots. It is unique in that it grows in symbiosis with a host tree. Mistletoe roots itself in the inner part of the stem or branches of trees. It has white fruit, small translucent beads that contain a single seed. This interesting plant has always been considered miraculous. The Druids, who were Celtic priests, associated mistletoe with the power of fire and lightning. The plant was so valuable that touching it with human hands was not allowed, and its harvesting was done with a golden sickle. In many parts of Europe, it was hung on the front door as protection from lightning and earthquakes. At Christmas time, it is a tradition in many parts of the world to kiss under the mistletoe to bring forth a happy and prosperous new year. But beware: all parts of the plant are toxic. If properly processed, it can be used as a phytopharmaceutical, but only under strict control.

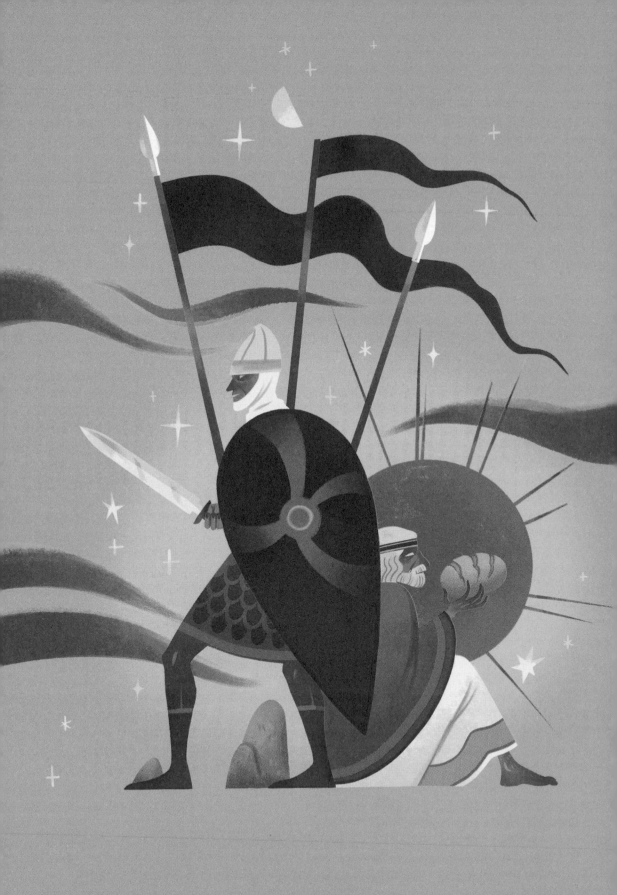

ACORN BREAD

Acorns, the fruit of the oak tree,
fall in large quantities.
If properly processed,
they can be turned into flour
to make an ancient
and magical bread.

Acorn-flour bread comes from the Norman tradition. Traces of it can be found in different parts of Italy, particularly in Sardinia, an island rich with oak trees. Acorn bread has been known since ancient times, and it is mentioned by Pliny the Elder in his *Naturalis Historia*. At that time, it was prepared by drying the acorns and treating them, then filtering the treated acorns with clay and ash to make unleavened bread that was baked either in the sun or in the oven.

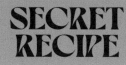

SECRET RECIPE

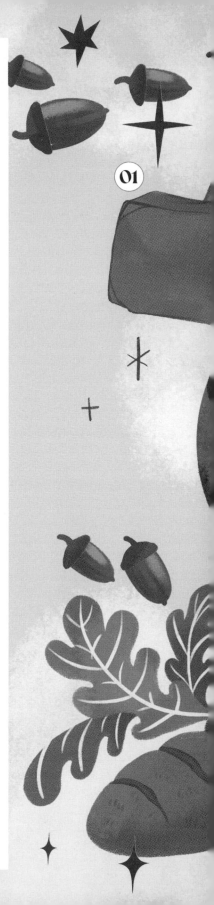

Acorns are high in protein and contain carbohydrates, fats, minerals, and vitamins. In particular, acorns have niacin, a vitamin that is lacking in grains. Mixing acorn flour with wheat flour makes for a more nutritionally complete food.

To knead the bread, dissolve the yeast in warm water, then slowly add the two flours, working them together **01**.

Let the dough rise for at least two hours or until it has doubled in volume **02**. Bake in a hot oven at 400°F (200 °C) for the first 15 minutes, then bake at 350°F (180°C) for the following 45–50 minutes **03**.

INGREDIENTS

- → **2 CUPS (250 G) ACORN FLOUR**
- → **6 CUPS (750 G) WHEAT FLOUR**
- → **1¼ CUPS (300 G) SOURDOUGH STARTER OR 2.5 TABLESPOONS BAKER'S YEAST**
- → **WATER, AS MUCH AS IS NEEDED**

ACORNS

Acorns are the fruit of the oak tree. Oak trees belong to the Fagaceae family, to which the chestnut tree also belongs. Acorns make up a large part of the diet of deer, bears, and wild boar, and are are edible for humans if properly treated. An ancient recipe for making acorn flour involves letting the acorns dry in the sun for at least two days after harvesting. Then, to remove the tannins that make the acorns bitter and inedible, the acorns must be placed in a bucket and covered with water. The water should be changed daily until it runs clear. The acorns can then be peeled, removing both the hard outer shell and the inner husk. Finally, the acorns are dried again in the sun before they are ground into flour. Carrying an acorn as an amulet increases fertility and power and is also believed to protect against lightning.

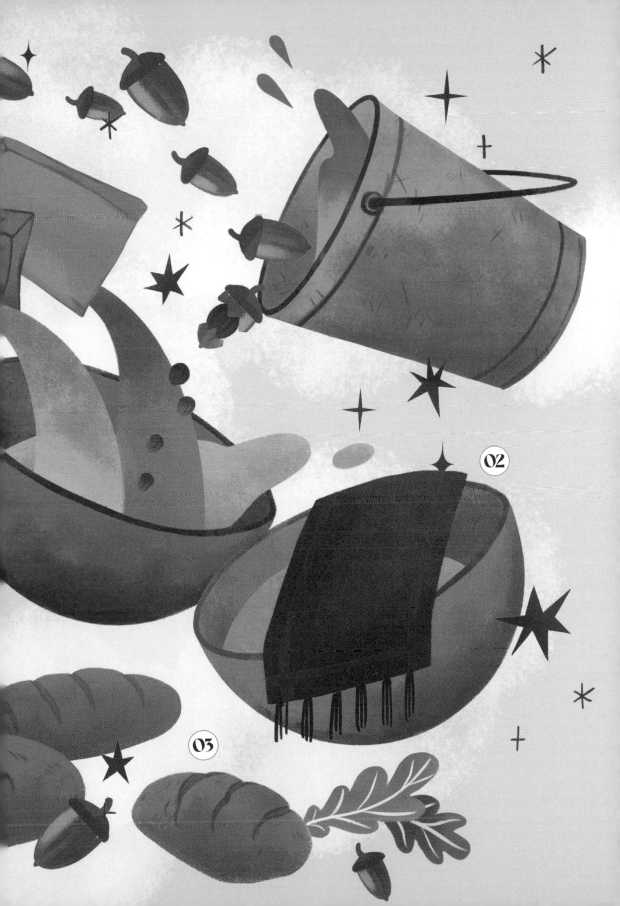

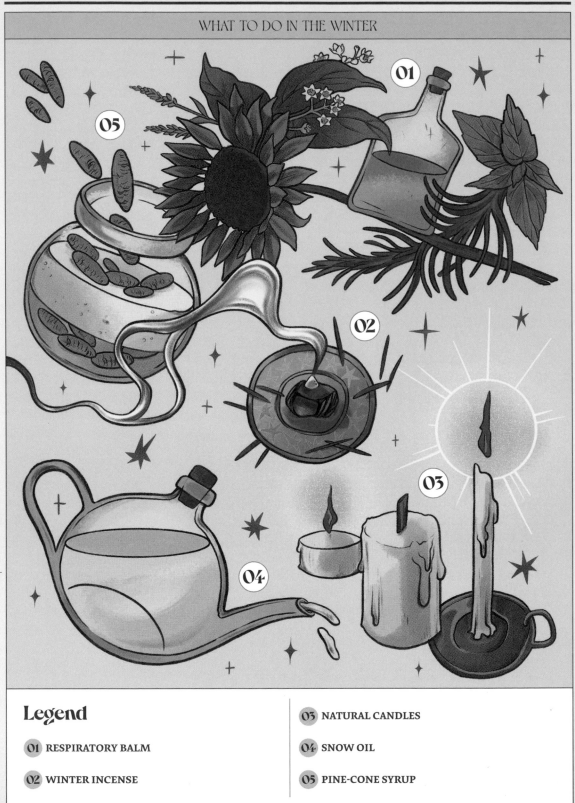

Legend

01 RESPIRATORY BALM

02 WINTER INCENSE

03 NATURAL CANDLES

04 SNOW OIL

05 PINE-CONE SYRUP

What to Do in the Winter

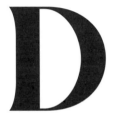uring the winter season, activities in the home are preferable, such as preparing a respiratory balm to let the soothing fragrance of the forest reach every corner of your lungs; gathering small pine cones from a bountiful pine tree to prepare cough remedies; and getting cozy, warming up, reading, and writing down plans and dreams for spring.

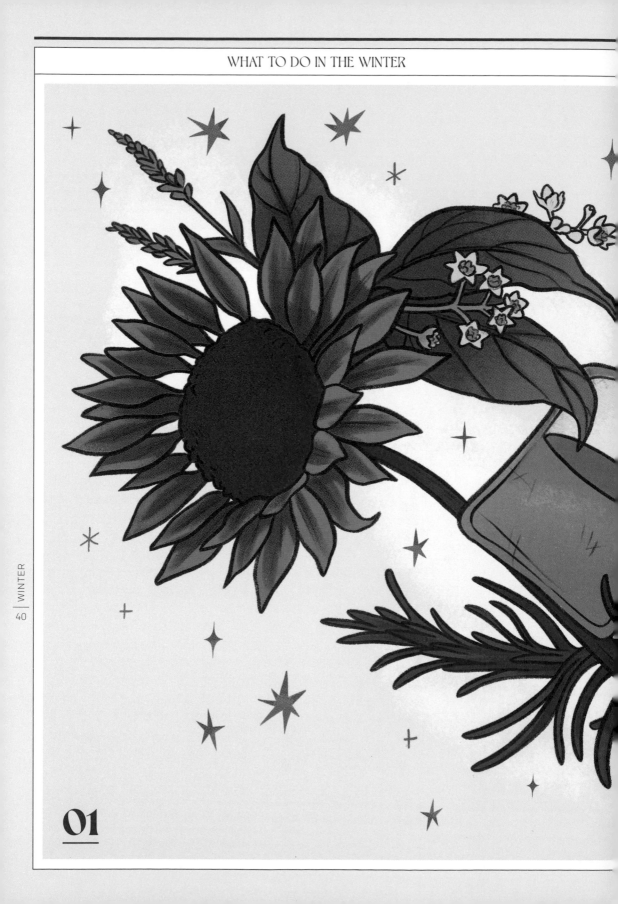

01

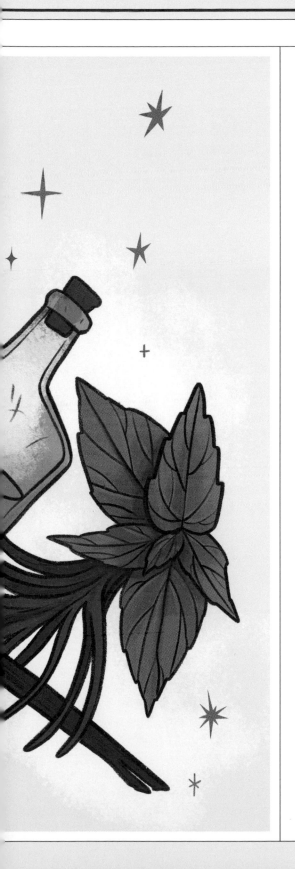

Respiratory Balm

You can prepare a respiratory balm to use for colds, nasal congestion, coughs, and other sicknesses. Melt 2 ounces (60 g) of sunflower oil, 1.4 ounces (40 g) of shea butter, and 0.3 ounces (10 g) of beeswax in a double boiler. Once these ingredients have melted together, remove from the pot and allow the mixture to cool slightly. Do not allow it to harden. Add 15 drops of mountain pine essential oil, 10 drops of mint essential oil, 5 drops of camphor essential oil, and 5 drops of lavender essential oil. Pour the mixture into a clean glass jar and let it cool. You can also use this balm on your temples if you have a headache.

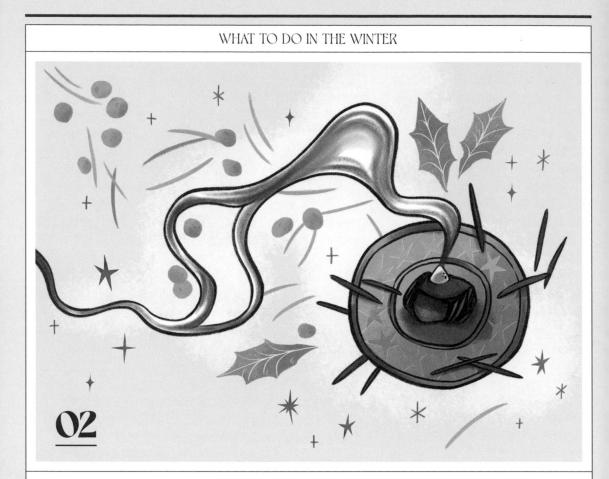

02

Winter Incense

During the long winter evenings, make incense by mixing dried resins and herbs. Burn incense by placing it on a small burning coal in a fireproof container. Put one part incense grains, two parts pine needles or resin, one part holly bark, and one part juniper cones in a mortar. Grind the ingredients, then store them in a container with a lid. You can burn a small amount of this incense to harmonize your energy with that of the winter season and to purify your home. To avoid excess smoke, burn incense only in well-ventilated rooms. Pine needles mixed with the pointed leaves of holly repel negativity, and the plants used in this mixture have refreshing and soothing properties that will purify the home on both physical and energetic levels.

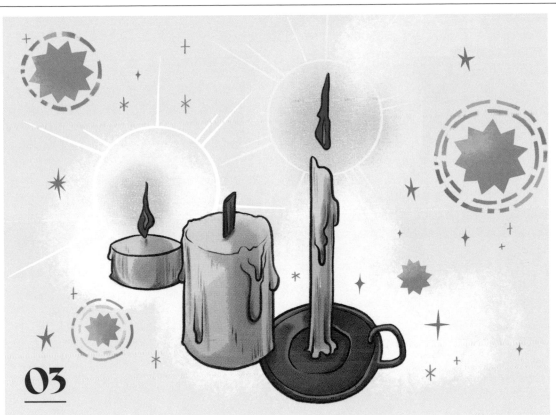

03

Natural Candles

Natural candles are simple to make. Their base is soy wax, a plant-based wax that does not release harmful substances once lit, as can happen with kerosene. Creating a natural candle can be a nice activity to engage in during the winter, to celebrate light even at the darkest time of the year. To do this, buy a loaf of soy wax, which you can find in herbalist shops or online. Melt 10 ounces (300 g) of soy wax in a double boiler. While the wax melts, prepare a glass jar into which you will pour your candle. You can use a wooden wick, which is a completely natural thin strip of wood attached to the wick holder and secured to the bottom of the container. (Wooden wicks are also available online.) Once the wax is melted, pour it into the jar, making sure that the wick remains in the center. You can decorate the candle with fir needles, juniper berries, and other winter plants. Once the wax has solidified, you can light your candle and celebrate the winter solstice!

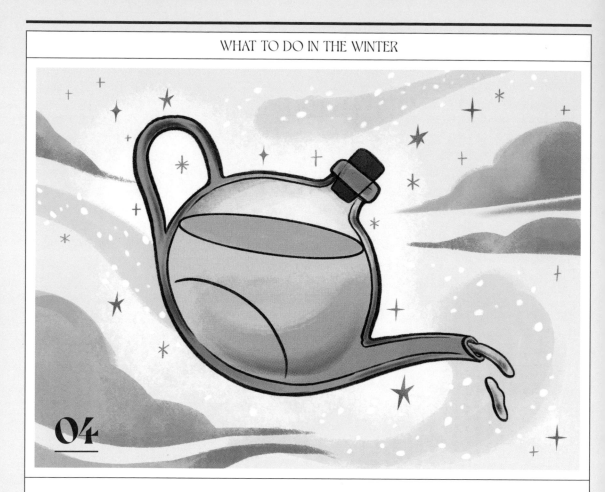

04

Snow Oil

This recipe for snow oil harkens back to ancient traditions. An herbana witch was handed down this recipe from a dear friend, who in turn had learned it from her grandmother. It is a simple, treasured recipe because it can only be prepared in winter, and only if we encounter snow. After a heavy snowfall, one must go to a place where the snow is clean. Collect the clean snow in a bowl then add olive oil slowly until you get a soft mixture. The mixture should be used right away; it does not keep well. It can be rubbed on red skin as a soothing agent or on irritated or rough body parts to soften and exfoliate. If you want, you can cover the application with clean gauze until completely absorbed. Snow oil is very special because it can only be prepared after a fresh winter snowfall and must be used immediately after it is made. It is an ancient remedy belonging to another time that has been passed down orally, making it a fascinating and useful tradition.

05

Pine-Cone Syrup

The right time to collect pine buds and their small pine cones is in the latter part of winter or early spring when the snow has receded. To make pine-cone syrup, collect cones and buds while they are still green and resiny. Take only enough to fill a glass jar. Alternate the small green pine cones and sugar in layers until the whole jar is filled. Shake it often, so that all the empty spaces between the pine cones are filled: if you want, you can add honey as well, making sure the contents of the jar are uniformly covered. Close the jar and leave it in the sun in front of the window or outside for at least three weeks. If you see that the sugar melts, leaving pine cones uncovered, add more sugar. After at least three weeks have passed, strain the syrup through gauze and store it in the refrigerator. Use it within a season for coughs, colds, or sore throats.

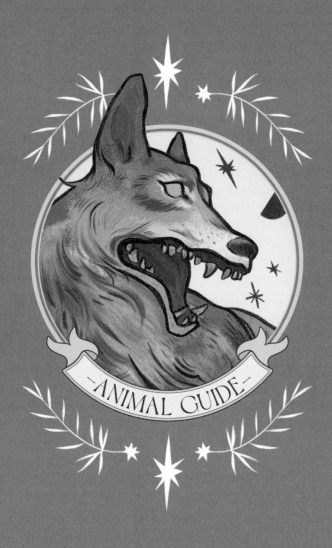

-ANIMAL GUIDE-

THE WOLF

The wolf is the animal
that best embodies
the wild spirit
of the forest.

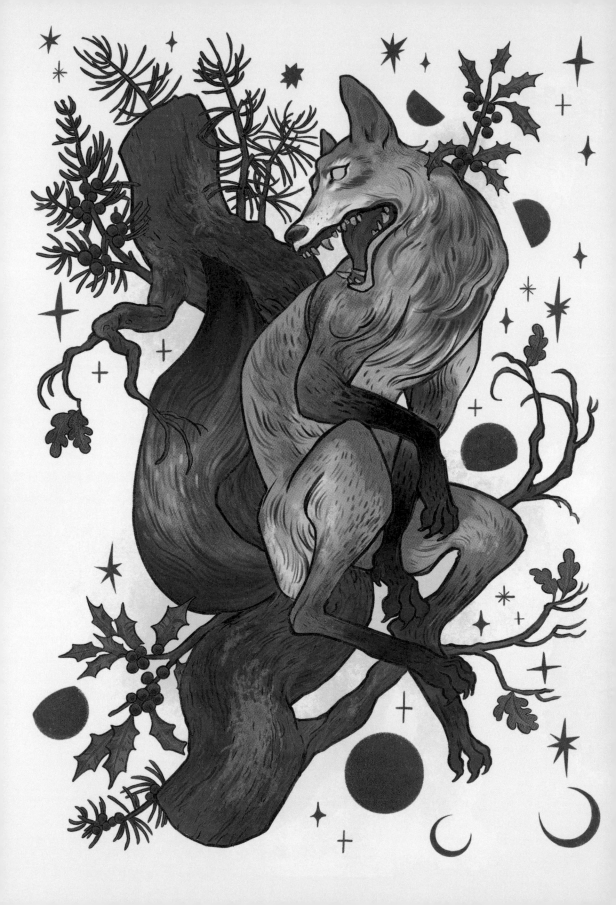

*Solitary yet part of a pack, **the wolf knows how to be both a leader and a follower**, but his spirit always remains intact. In fairy tales, **he often embodies mystery**, **the unknown**, or **the sacred**. Because he is linked to initiation, the wolf presides over winter, which is an initiation for us into spring and rebirth.*

THE WOLF stops at the edge of the forest and observes. He is not so different from dogs—a human's best friend—but at the same time, he is unfamiliar, wild, leading us to an unknown place. His ability to blend in has often led humans to associate him with the threshold and the spirit world. To the Celts, he was a lunar animal. Every evening, he would devour the sun to allow the moon to shine. This lunar nature makes him ambiguous, something which is evident in the fact that he belongs to both the world of instincts, embodying its highest expression, and to the world of reason, because of his connection with the pack and spirit of protection. In some traditions, the wolf brings light. For example, Odin, a Norse deity, is shown accompanied by two wolves, and the door to Valhalla is built of wolf skin. The wolf penetrates the darkness with its gaze. It is also a nocturnal animal and an expert predator.

For the Etruscans and ancient Egyptians, the wolf was the one who accompanied souls to the afterlife. The Egyptian god Anubis, who presided over necropolises, had the head of a jackal, an animal belonging to the same genus as the wolf.

Light and shadow, life and death alternate in the definition of this splendid animal. The herbana witch considers both aspects and knows that she walks on the edge between known and unknown, just like the wolf. The wolf and the herbana witch know each other. Perhaps, in a secret place in the woods, they meet, speaking the mysterious language that connects all living things.

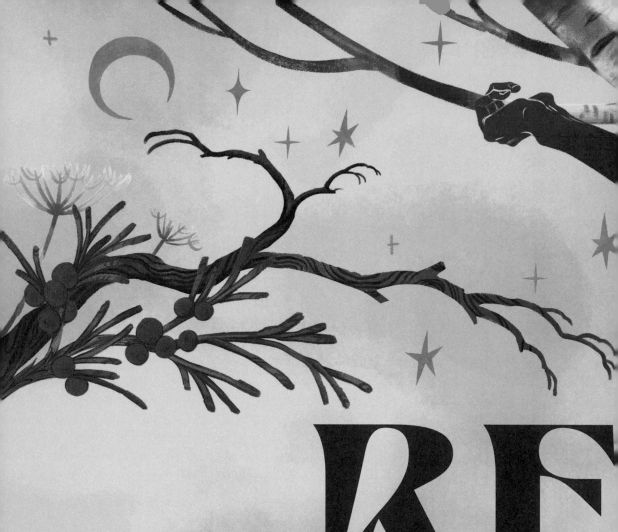

RE

THE HERBANA WITCH'S MESSAGE

In winter, do as the forest does: rest. Give yourself long breaks, find moments in your daily life to decompress, let go of your thoughts freely, laze about. It is important to stay still without doing anything, to rest. In a consumerist society, rest is not viewed positively. We see this attitude in stores that are open 24/7, fervent business activities that continue even into weekends, and the drive to do without ever stopping. Winter can inspire you to go in the opposite direction: to stop, slow down, regenerate. Seek stillness,

ST

in your soul and in your environment. Waste time. Dream a lot, especially daydreaming. Rest is necessary to fuel moments of activity, to find new ideas, which almost always come from a fertile void. Be like the seed in the ground, dreaming while waiting for the right time to germinate. Don't fear emptiness, the long nights. Let the sun, which retreats in the winter, guide you. Favor sleep and inactivity. For once, try doing one less thing instead of one more. Stubbornly practice slowness, and marvel at what you discover.

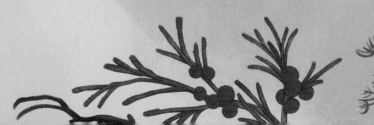

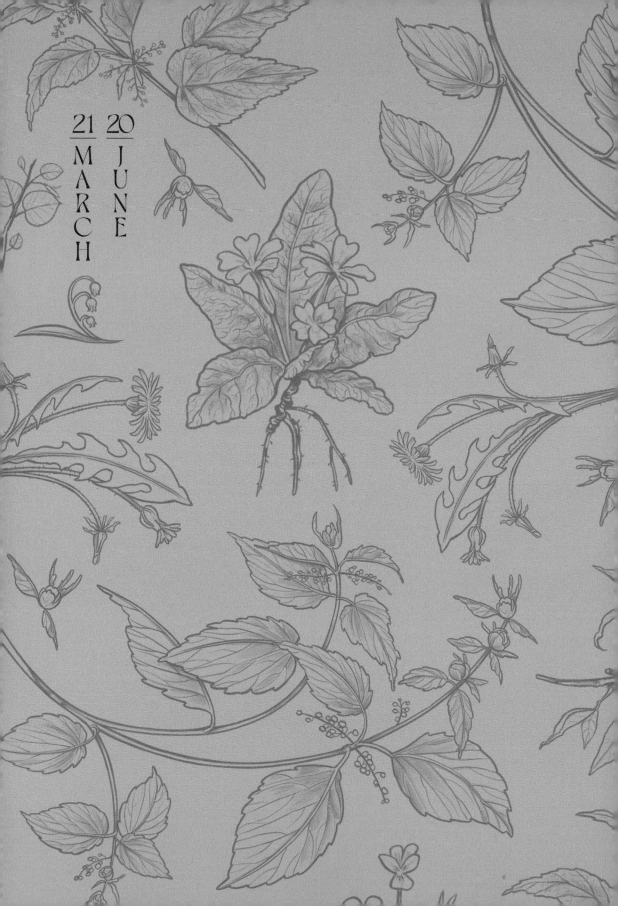

21 MARCH

20 JUNE

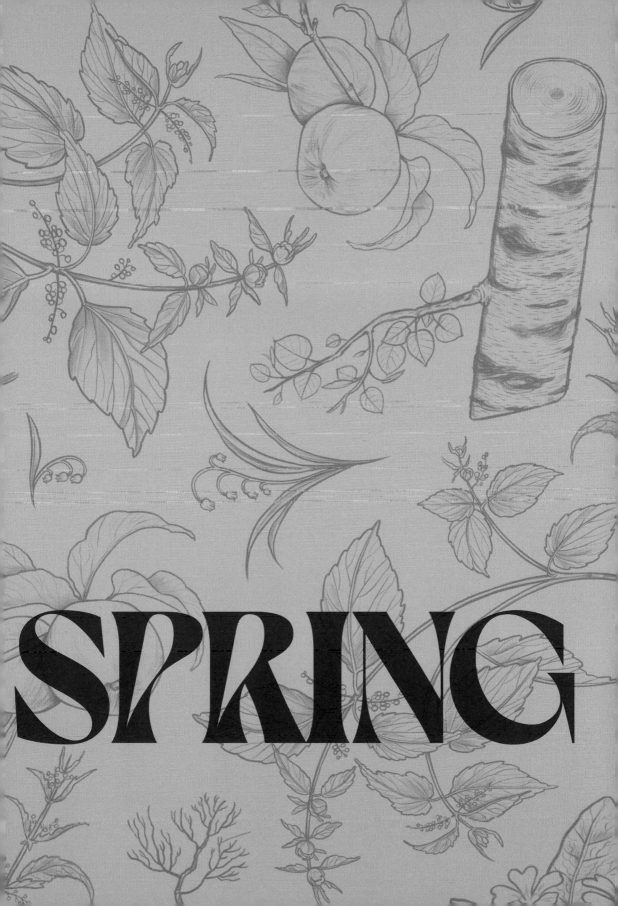

SPRING

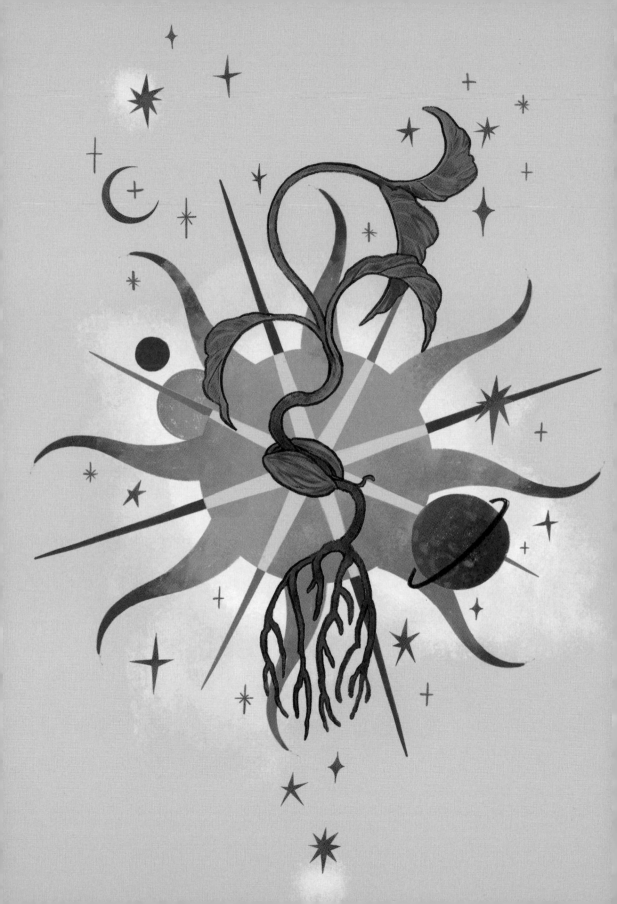

This is the time of the sprout, which contains the impetus of life that is just beginning.

The sprout is the part of the plant that is linked to the imagination and its ability to plan, create, and transform. It is the blade of grass breaking through the soil, the tale of the future. Through observing the sprout, we see the unfolding seedling is a reflection of our ability to open ourselves up, give ourselves to others, or to close ourselves off and focus on ourselves and our interiority. From plant sprouts, we can extract what is called a "bud-derivate," which is a glyceric macerate that is taken orally and contains the whole plant with its full beneficial potential.
Observe the buds of the trees you encounter every day. Stop to listen and you will know whether you must stay open or closed, turn outward or inward. If you look closely, a bud can resemble an egg: the synthesis of creation, closed but permeable, ready to be born with new life.

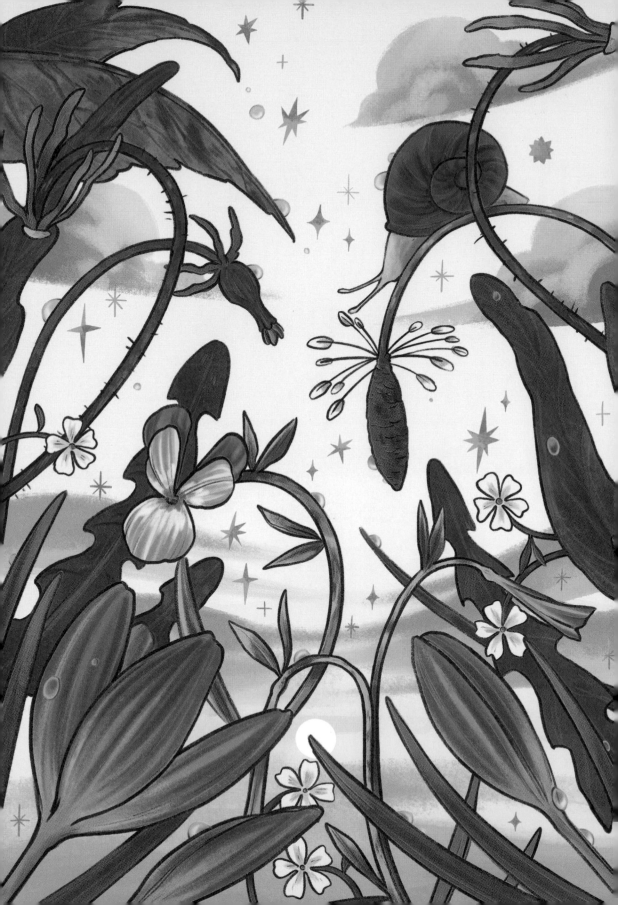

The herbana witch knows that spring is coming when the crocuses sprout.

Like tiny plant fireworks, they pop up here and there, discreetly at first, before they paint the edges of paths or clearings under chestnut trees with purple. After that come the primroses (*Primula veris*) and the violets (*Viola odorata*), the former being exuberant and explosive with their bright colors and fleshy leaves; the latter more reserved and introverted, reflecting the mysteries of the season and preserving them in the depths of their dark purple color. This is the time of the year when, every morning, as soon as the dew dries on the leaves and petals, one must go out with a basket and scissors to gather wild edible herbs: dandelion (*Taraxacum officinale*), nettle (*Urtica dioica*), the first plantain leaves (*Plantago major* or *lanceolata*), and a few honesty flowers (*Lunaria annua*) to decorate salads and risottos.

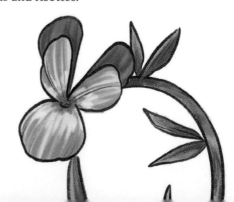

In winter, when the forest is silent and seemingly asleep, we experience emptiness. It is precisely because of the space created in winter, the rest and reflection, that it is now possible to be reborn, renewed with energy. The herbana witch knows that this is a good time to clean the house, throw away herbs more than a year old, and prepare pots and small containers for seedlings that will be transplanted into the garden in May. She knows that this is the time of year when the air becomes sweeter, the full moon shines with a golden glow, and animals, sensing that everything is awakening and renewed, begin to seek out each other.

Spring is the season of Aphrodite. The Rosaceae plants dedicated to her, like roses and apple trees, have crimson flowers streaked with white and pink that seem to beckon for love. It is time to clean up, renew our connections and relationships, learn to be light-hearted, which is not the same as superficiality. It is the beauty of the everyday, the power in simplicity.

We read spring as if it were a new tale every year, one we can remember only by the colors of the flowers. Even the evening in spring becomes sweeter, and the day stretches toward the twilight, into the indigo sky. The robins have finished their nests and the young beech trees have bright green leaves. They look like an idea formed by stars in the evening dusk. Our hearts become lighter, for beauty speaks to us, accompanies us through this season, and teaches us the power of being here and now, just like the sprouts, perfect in their being before they flower.

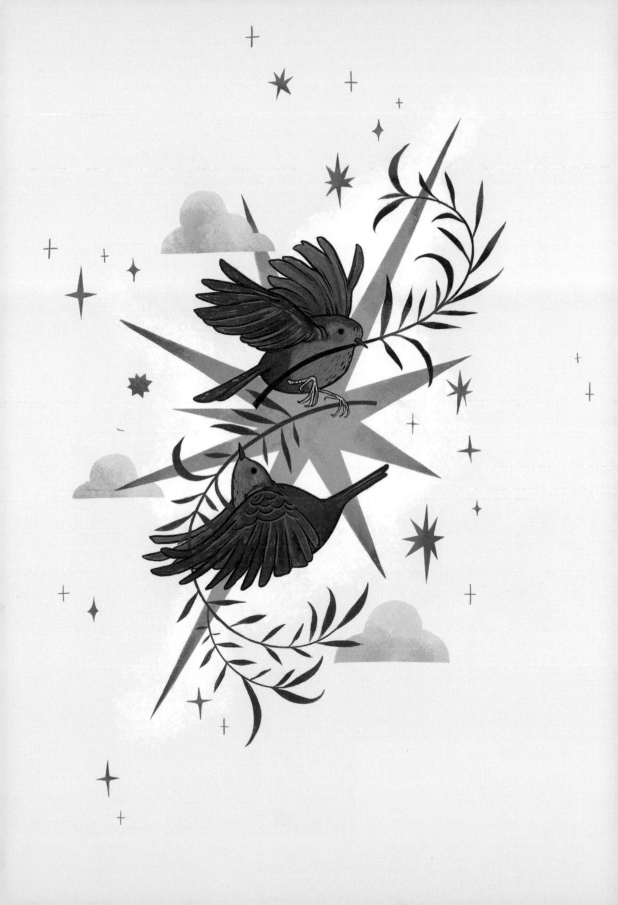

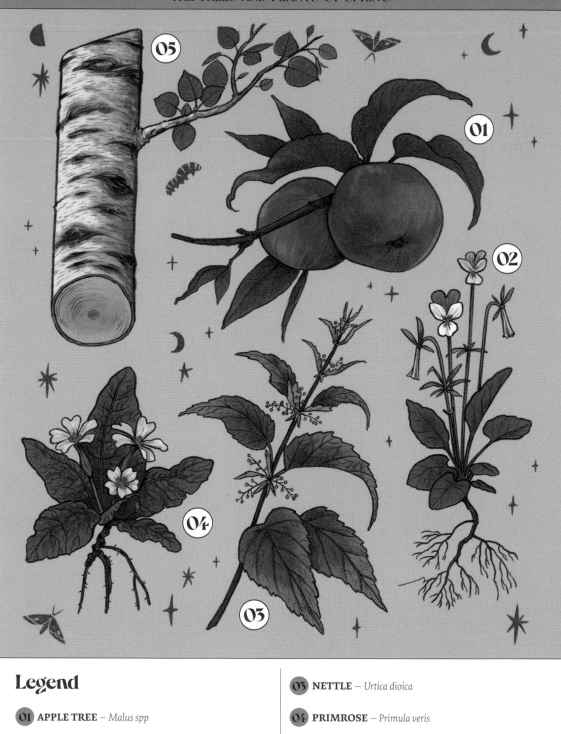

Legend

01 **APPLE TREE** – *Malus spp*

02 **VIOLET** – *Viola odorata*

03 **NETTLE** – *Urtica dioica*

04 **PRIMROSE** – *Primula veris*

05 **BIRCH** – *Betula alba*

The Trees and Plants of Spring

When spring arrives, you can tell by little signs: the trees fill with buds, the green of the leaves becomes brighter, the scent in the air becomes fresh and herbaceous. As the sun begins to warm, it's nice to take a few breaks from daily activities and stand under its rays. We feel everything around us begin to wake up from the slumber of winter.

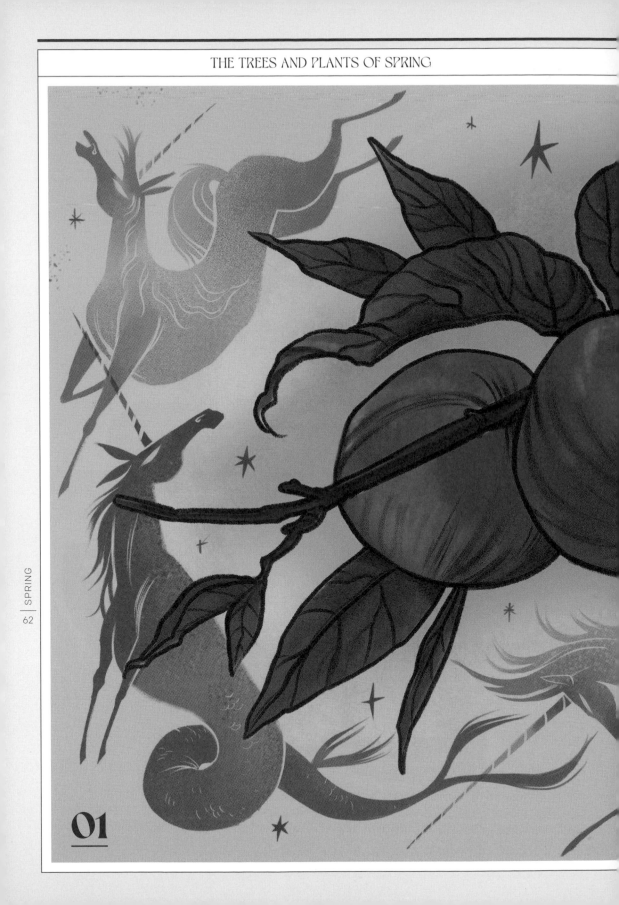

01

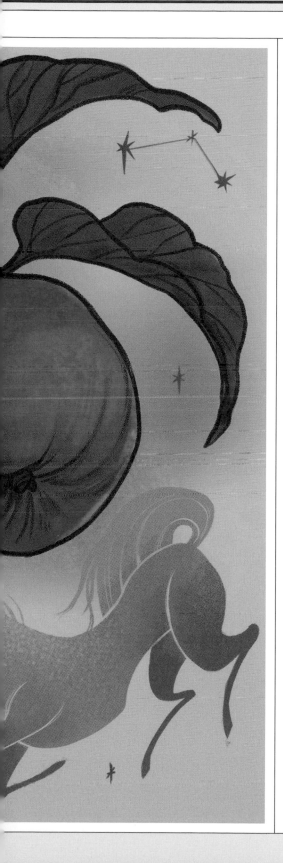

Apple Tree

The flowers of the apple tree seem enchanted. Pink and white, they open joyfully in spring. It's no coincidence that the sacred plant of the island of Avalon, the land of the priestess in Arthurian mythology, was an apple tree. The apple, a plant dedicated to Venus, is in the same family as the rose. It is an expression of love and purity. The apple tree is a symbol of beginnings, signified by the very first tree in the Garden of Eden. The fruit of the apple tree holds a secret. If cut horizontally, its seeds form a star, a symbol of the five elements (earth, air, water, fire, and spirit), which connects this plant to natural magic. The flowers of the crapabble tree can be used to make one of Dr. Bach's remedies for promoting love for your authentic self. With healing, attention, and love toward ourselves, we can restore beauty and harmony to the world and bring paradise back to earth. Wood from the apple tree can be used to make your magic wand, especially if you feel a strong connection to fairies. Lastly, it is said that unicorns are attracted to apple trees in the spring.

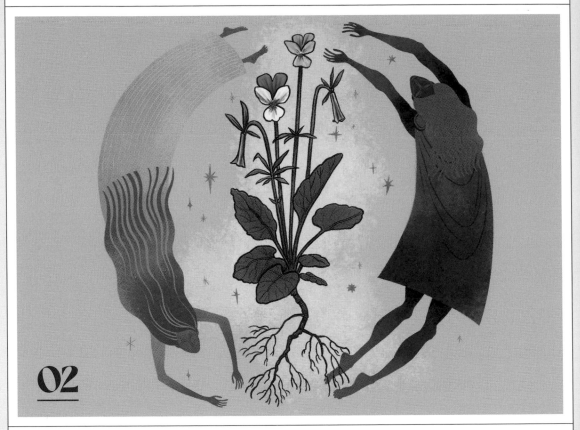

02

Violet

Myth has it that fragrant violets were born under the footsteps of Persephone, goddess of spring, who ascended to Earth after the winter months ended. Violets are recognizable by their heart-shaped leaves and unmistakably purple and fragrant, soft little flowers. The herbana witch uses all parts of the plant: the leaves can be eaten raw and have a refreshing taste; the flowers, which are also edible, can be used to decorate cakes, salads, or ice cubes for drinks. Syrup made from violet flowers is very popular with children both for its flavor and its intense, fairy-like pink color. Violet has expectorant properties: it relieves dry coughs and is refreshing and emollient. It also has depurative properties, helping the body eliminate excessive heat and toxins retained by the liver. In folk tradition, a wreath of violet flowers soothes headaches and violets are used along with rose, lavender, yarrow, and apple blossom in herbal teas for self-love. Its leaves are said to keep evil away.

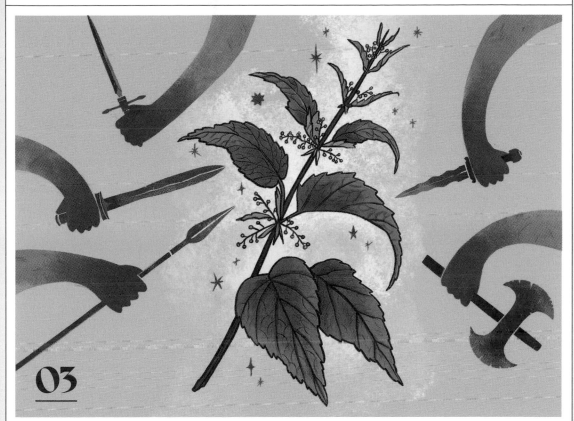

03

Nettle

An herbana witch knows that in order to fully bloom, it is necessary to establish specific personal boundaries. This is the message of nettle, which grows wild everywhere these days, especially in iron-rich soils. If at first glance it seems to you that all green plants look alike, nettle teaches that this is not the case. Try touching it, and you will recognize it immediately! Nettle leaves have tiny needles containing formic acid, which break when touched, causing its famous stinging sensation. Rich in vitamins and minerals, nettle is beneficial for our blood. It regenerates hemoglobin and promotes iron absorption. Connected to Mars, nettle is energizing and restorative. The little green warrior knows how to set boundaries and give itself generously. Risotto with nettle is a delicious specialty of the herbana witch's table in spring. Nettle roots worn in a red pouch protect against negative energy. Burning dried nettle leaves as incense drives away stagnant energy and protects the home.

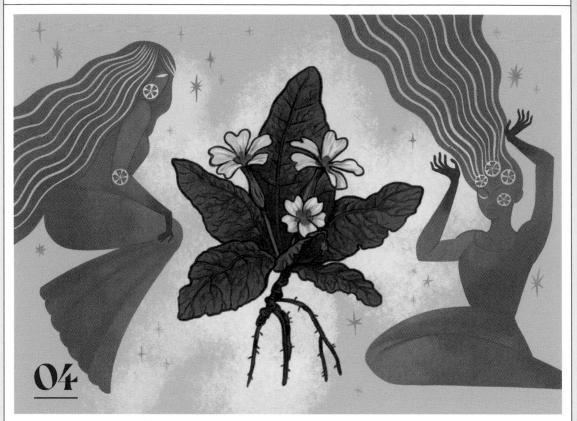

04

Primrose

The primrose is one of the flowers that heralds spring. With its colorful, sun-yellow flowers, it is a symbol of prosperity, good luck, and well-being. In the past, primrose was used to make a variety of herbal teas; its leaves for rheumatism and its roots as a migraine soother. Folk medicine recommends primrose flower infusion not only for headaches but also as an expectorant and fever reducer, due to the salicylic acid in the seedling. You can use primrose flowers as decorative additions to salads or herbal teas, and even on bread and cookies. In Italy, *Primula veris* is a protected species. You can pick *Primula vulgaris* flowers instead, which have the same properties, albeit milder. Putting a primrose flower in your mouth is said to help you see fairies, and holding a bunch of primroses in your hand is a great charm for when you need to find hidden treasure. Planting primrose outside your front door or keeping it in a pot keeps unwanted visitors away.

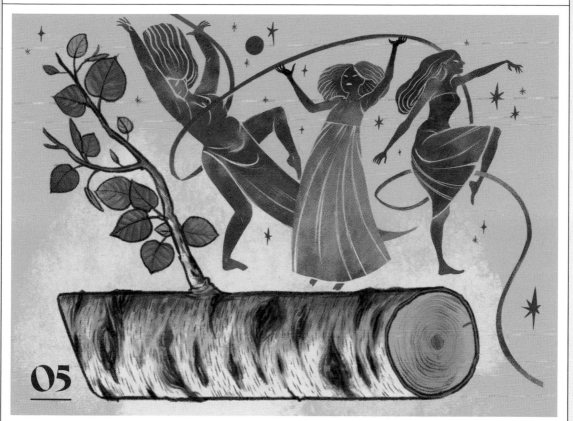

05

Birch

The birch has been associated with spring since Celtic times. For the Celts, it was a symbol of renewal, death, and rebirth. It holds the ability to become a threshold, to preside over the realm of the dead as well as festivals related to life and fertility. Beltane rites were celebrated in groves of birch trees, and the bodies of the deceased were covered with birch branches in Celtic funeral rites. The *Berkana* rune, which looks like a "b," takes its name from this tree and means renewal or rebirth. The birch coincides with the power of spring, which, in order to express itself, must first make room. The birch is a pioneer tree. It repopulates the land after a fire, to prepare it for new plant and animal settlements. Birch is mainly used for detoxing, whether through its sap, which is an excellent remedy for a cleanse after the winter months, or as an herbal tea made from its leaves. Birch bud-derivate is also one of the primary detox agents used in bud-therapy.

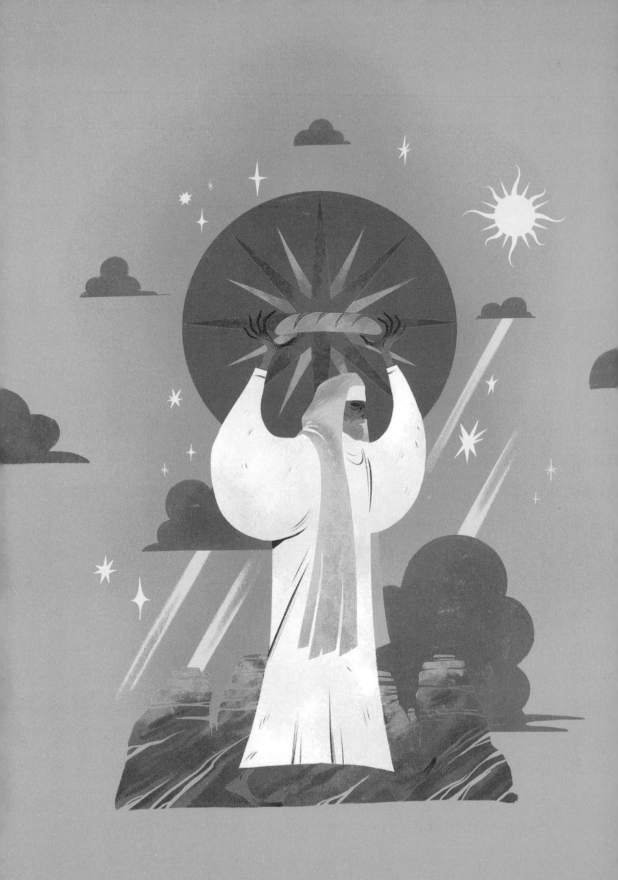

BREAD WITH SPROUTS AND SEEDS

To celebrate spring, the herb witch bakes a beautiful bread with a very ancient tradition. It is a special bread made without flour. Instead, sprouted grains and oily seeds are used.

This particular recipe dates back to the second century BCE, when the Essenes, a Jewish monastic group, began making it using grain that had sprouted after threshing and remained on the ground waiting to be gathered. This very special bread is made by sprouting wheat kernels for about 12 to 24 hours, then blending them and mixing them with oily seeds. The baking of this bread is also special. It is done at a low temperature to prevent damaging the properties of the sprouts. Sprouted wheat has many properties: it is rich in antioxidants, B vitamins, folic acid, and fiber.

DIFFICULTY: EASY

SECRET RECIPE

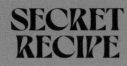

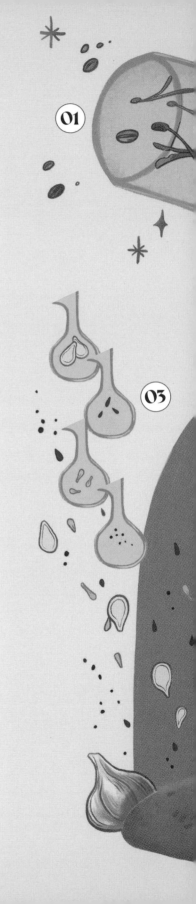

You will need 17 ounces (500 g) of grain: wheat, oats, or barley are fine for this recipe **01**. You will need to sprout them for 12 to 24 hours. Once they are sprouted, you can blend them together with four tablespoons of extra virgin olive oil and some lukewarm water—but not so much that it makes the mixture too liquid **02**. At this point, you can add a few tablespoons of oily seeds: sunflower seeds, pumpkin seeds, poppy seeds, or flax seeds are fine. They will add taste and nutrition to this already very digestible and nutritious bread **03**. Create small loaves from the dough, then flatten the loaves to a height of about one centimeter, a little less than one half inch. **04**. Bake them, preferably, in a dehydrator or a convection oven set at 120–160°F (50–70°C) until they are crumbly. Brush the surface of the bread with garlic water (made by soaking a few cloves of minced garlic in water for about ten minutes) and your bread will keep even longer.

INGREDIENTS

→ **3¼ CUPS (500 G) GRAINS (WHEAT, OATS, BARLEY)**
→ **4 TABLESPOONS EXTRA VIRGIN OLIVE OIL**
→ **FEW TABLESPOONS OILY SEEDS**
  (SUNFLOWER, PUMPKIN, POPPY, FLAX)

SPROUTS AND SPROUTING

Making sprouts—from seeds, grains, or legumes—at home is simple and inexpensive. You need:
- seeds to sprout, which you can find in bags in any store;
- a sprouter, or a glass container (a jar or bowl) that allows air to circulate;
- a lid that allows the water to drain, a mesh covering attached to the jar with a rubber band, or paper towels which can be removed and replaced when rinsing.

Let the seeds soak overnight, then put them in the jar and rinse them twice a day. It is important when rinsing that no water remains. Be sure to remove all of it or drain the seeds with a colander. After three or four days, they will be ready! Store your sprouts in the refrigerator and add them to salads, croutons, juices, and so on.

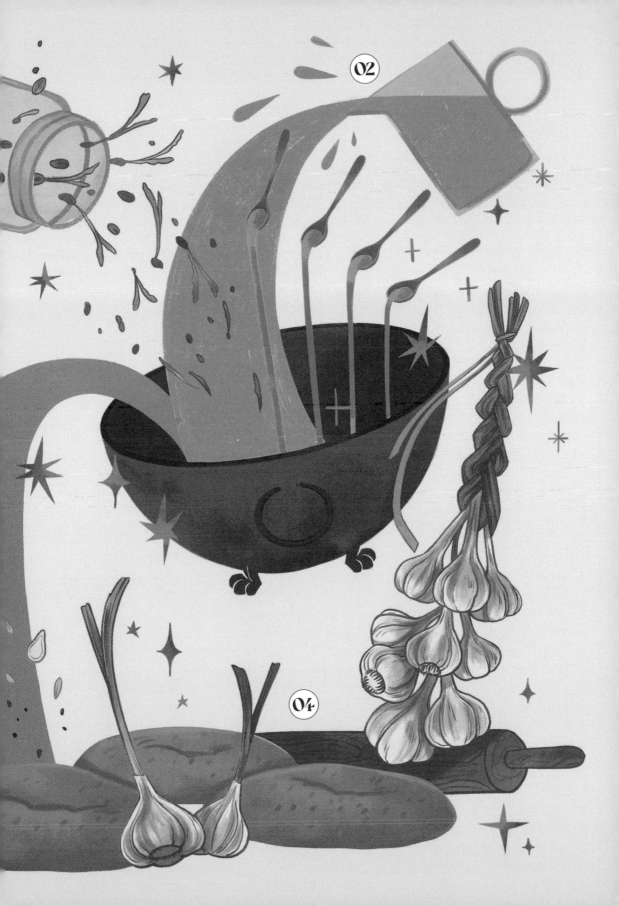

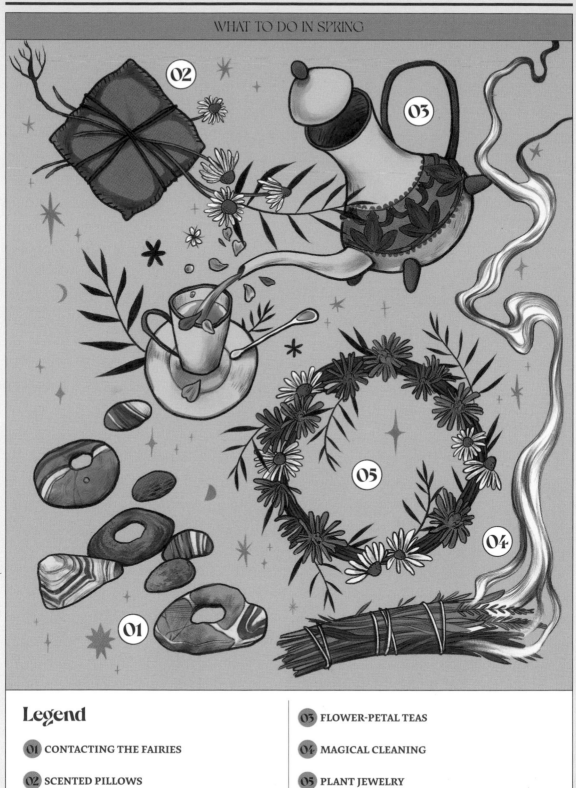

Legend

01 CONTACTING THE FAIRIES

02 SCENTED PILLOWS

03 FLOWER-PETAL TEAS

04 MAGICAL CLEANING

05 PLANT JEWELRY

What to Do in Spring

The herbana witch's house shines in the spring after her magical cleaning process. Her seedlings are lush, the prism in the window casts dancing rainbows, and if you look closely you will see a fairy or two speeding by in the wild back garden. This is the best season to make little scented pillow-amulets, to magically clean your house, and to contact the fairies, the most elusive of the Wee Folk. This is the best time of year to renew, refresh, bloom, and clean. In spring, we too do as the seedlings do: sprout up with new life under the soft March sun.

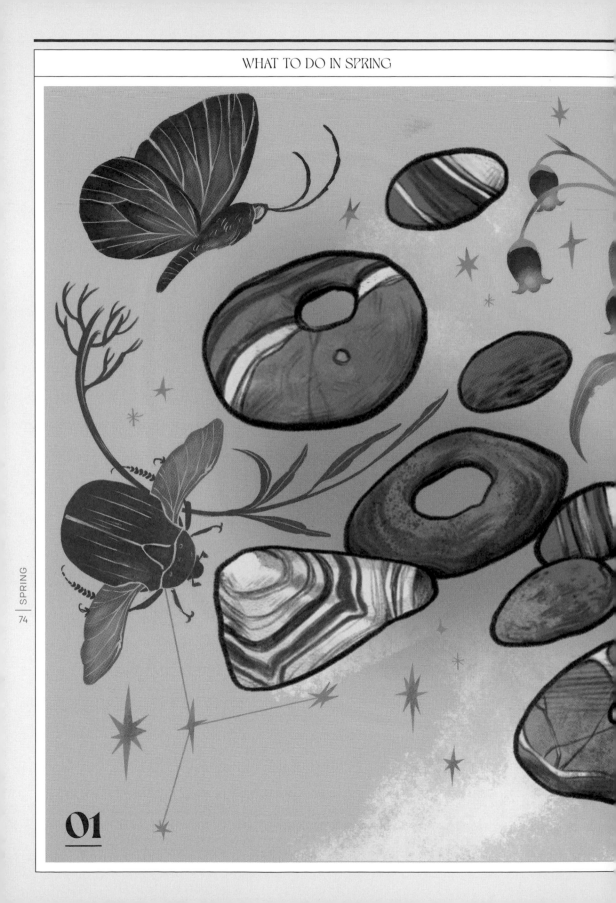

01

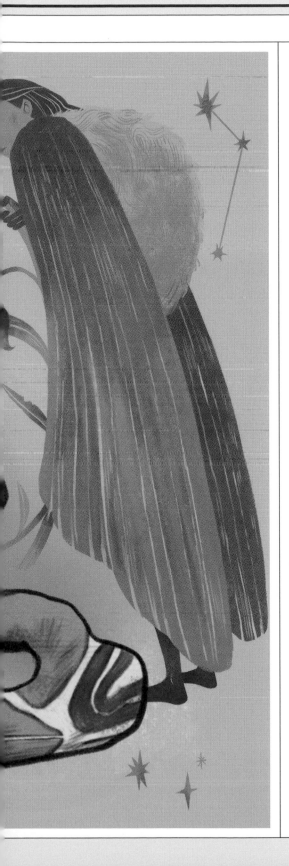

Contacting the Fairies

Fairies are around in every season, but in spring, if you are lucky, you can contact them the most easily. Remember that they do not like to be disturbed, and you will have to be patient and move discreetly. One way to see fairies is to taste a primrose flower. If you encounter wild primroses on one of your walks, try eating one or two of the little flowers. They are rich in salicylic acid and very sugary (remember that it is essential to be able to correctly identify a plant before eating it). Stones with holes are magical objects that are said to grant people the power to see the invisible. If you find a pierced stone and look through it, you might spot a fairy. Another way to spot one is to take care of a natural space without intervening too much. Remember to leave a part of your garden, balcony, or windowsill a little uncultivated. This will be a haven for the little fairy creatures that pass by your house. The fairies will thank you silently, without your seeing them.

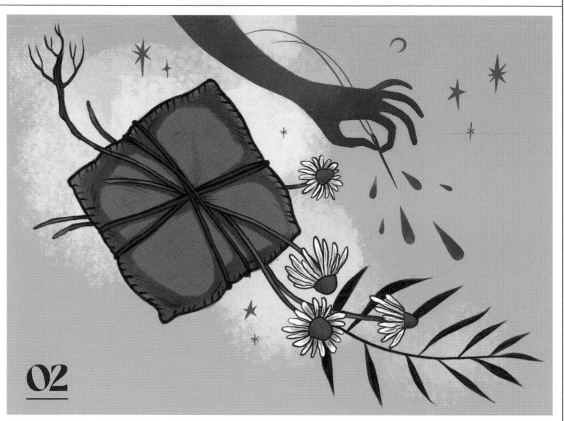

02

Scented Pillows

To make an herb-and-flower pillow, I recommend collecting fresh flowers and wild herbs, such as lemon balm, mint, chamomile, and poppy petals. Get two sheets of natural fabric measuring 6x4 inches (15x20 cm) each. You can choose them in a neutral color, dye them with herbal dyes (see the section on summer), or decide on a color you like that relaxes you. Once you have gathered the herbs and flowers, hang them upside down to dry in small bunches. Meanwhile, sew the three sides of the fabric together, remembering to turn the fabric inside out. Then turn it back outside in and stuff the pillow with the herbs and petals. You can also insert some cotton wool, cotton, or leftover stuffing from other pillows to make it thicker. If you like, add a few drops of the essential oil of your choice. Now sew the last side or install a zipper. You can add a small bell, a pierced stone, or a shell as a decoration. Here's a little secret: if you add mugwort leaves into the pillow, you might have prophetic dreams.

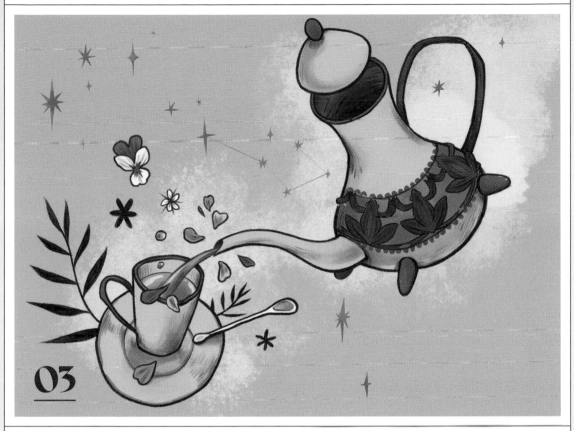

03

Flower-Petal Teas

To celebrate spring, prepare an herbal tea made entirely of flowers. It is best if you pick them yourself, but you can also buy them dried at an herbalist shop. Flowers are very delicate; unlike seeds, roots, or bark, they should be left to steep for less time, 5 to 10 minutes at most. Your spring herbal tea might consist of: a handful of mallow flowers (*Malva sylvestris*), a handful of poppy petals (*Papaver roehas*), two tablespoons of elderberry flowers (*Sambucus nigra*), a tablespoon of marigold flowers (*Calendula officinalis*), dandelion petals (*Taraxacum officinalis*), and borage flowers (*Borago officinalis*) for decoration. The water used to brew your tea should be pure, clear, colorless, and soft. Keep it at a temperature below 215°F (100°C) to prevent damage to the flowers. Bring it to a boil and then let it cool a few minutes. The doses given are good for 2 cups (0.5 l) of water. Here's a little secret: freeze the borage flowers inside ice cubes and use them to slightly cool the water. Sweeten with honey, if you like.

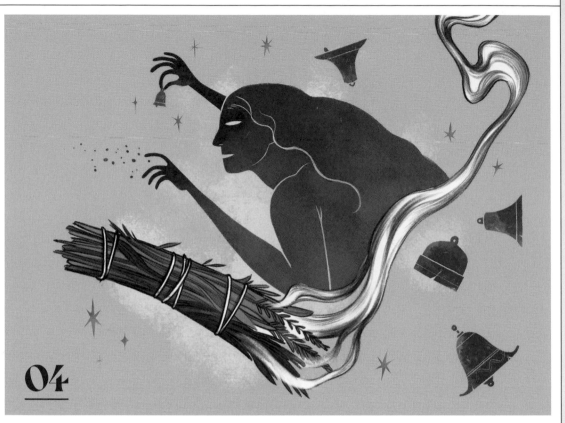

04

Magical Cleaning

In spring, find the time to magically clean your house just like any herbana witch. Start by opening the windows wide and airing out the rooms. You can light a stick of palo santo, an herb bundle of juniper, or incense such as thyme, mint, or lavender. Go through each area of your house, watching as the smoke exits through the windows, taking with it all that is stagnant and old. Prepare an infusion of mugwort and lavender and dissolve it in water to clean the floors. Add a few drops of tea tree essential oil to the mixture and mop each room. Put a few grains of rock salt in the corners of each room; rock salt has symbolic powers of protection and purification. Take a broom and sweep all the heavy energy you feel out the windows, visualizing it as a dark fog that gradually clears. Conclude your magical cleaning by ringing a little bell in each room.

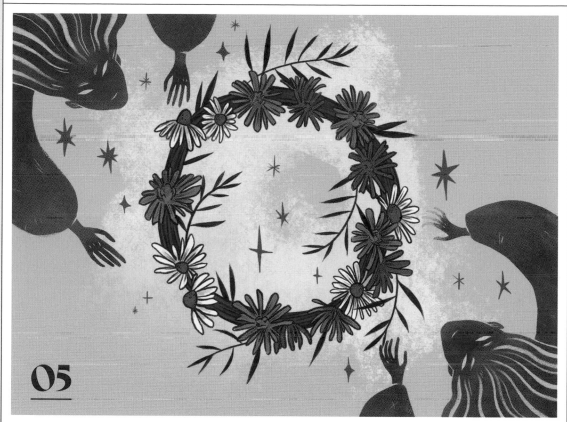

05

Plant Jewelry

Ephemeral jewelry made from flowers and plants is a splendid way to get in touch with spring. You can crown yourself king or queen of the woods for an afternoon by carefully gathering a few plant parts and creating a crown, necklace, or bracelet of flowers and leaves. Plant jewelry is very simple to make: bring along some soft wire to form a skeleton for your creation (a necklace or bracelet is suitable), and weave flowers, vines, twigs, and leaves until you have created a suitable sense of harmony. To create a wreath, weave together several bundles of soft twigs (broom, hazelnut, or ivy are perfect for this) and use wire to keep the plant and decorations in place. Wrap ribbons around the wires to hide them. Measure the width of your head with the wire so you get a proper fit for the wreath. Leave about 1 inch (3 cm) of room, then cut the wire, holding the ends in place with tape.

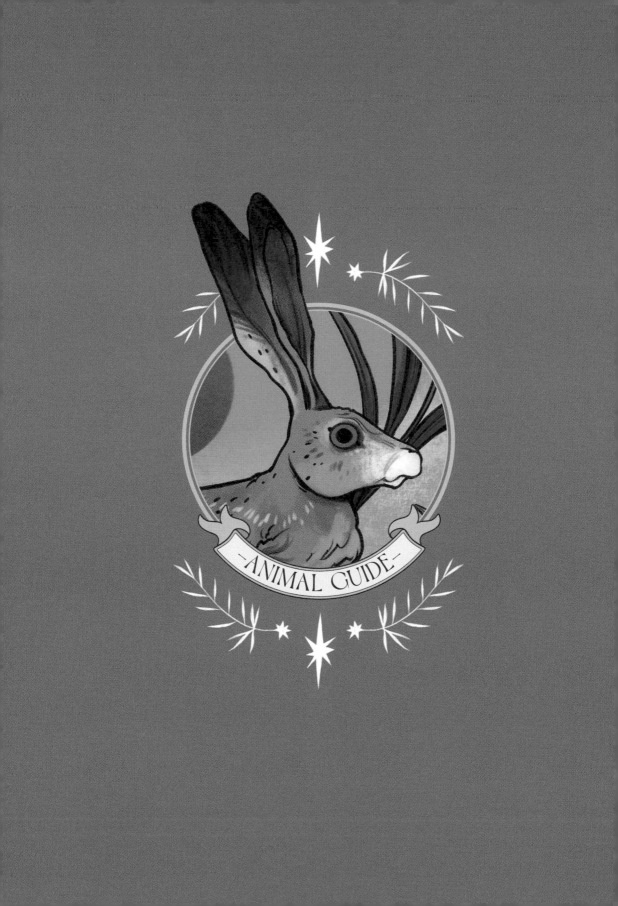

ANIMAL GUIDE

THE HARE

A symbol of fertility
and regeneration, the hare,
particularly the white hare,
is closely associated
with the return of spring.

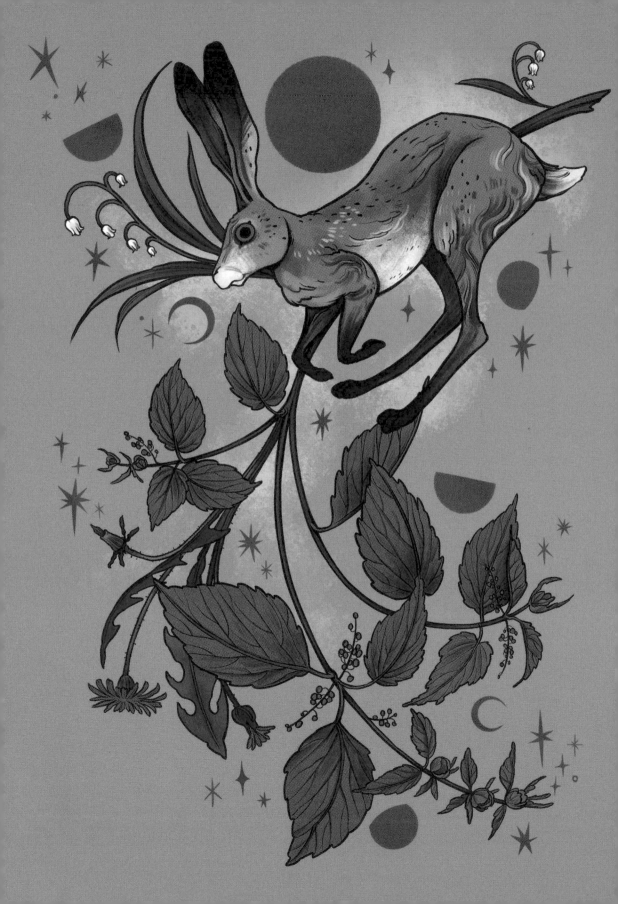

Hares and rabbits are often conflated, but in fact they are different. Hares live longer than rabbits and have dark coloring on their longer ears. **The hare is an animal associated with fertility and moon goddesses** *in the Greek world,* **like Aphrodite and Artemis**. *The hare was also used as a symbol by the Celts, Egyptians, and Native Americans.*

THE HARE is a nocturnal animal, hence its association with the moon and why we often find it depicted in nighttime settings. This link between the hare and the moon has inspired many myths. In China, Mexico, and Japan it is said that the moon looks like the profile of a hare. The full moon is a symbol of fertility, abundance, nourishment, and light, just like the hare. In Siberian mythology, Kaltes, goddess of the moon, often shows herself in the form of a hare. She is the goddess who protects birth and the beginning of life. In the Celtic world, the hare was often represented in threes to symbolize the cycle of life, death, and rebirth. The hare is a very fast animal. It lives on the edge, between the forest and countryside, and the speed with which it appears and disappears makes it a symbol of quick messages and intelligence.

It is often interpreted as a *trickster*, a figure that brings good luck but also creates surprises. That is the reason why the March Hare is found with the Mad Hatter in *Alice's Adventures in Wonderland*; Lewis Carroll did not put him there by accident. In spring, the hare's attitude is considered "crazy." Female hares that are not receptive to mating drive away males in a practice that resembles a boxing match. Meeting a hare means that something new, fresh, and unexpected is coming into our lives. We have the ability to move forward, to make ourselves independent and welcome the future. The hare reminds us not to take things too seriously, otherwise we will be deceived. We must stay open and welcoming in order to accept what is coming.

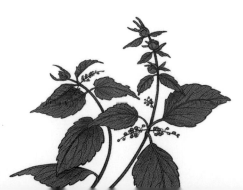

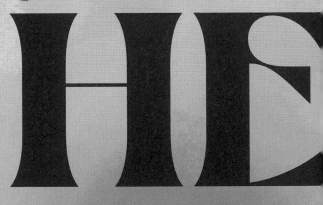

HE

THE HERBANA WITCH'S MESSAGE

Step into spring with all your senses alert. Taste what you eat and pay attention to the scents you encounter. Linger for a moment when touching coffee beans or the first basil and mint leaves. Lend your ear to birdsong. Observe carefully and consider the details. Try to look even where there seems to be nothing. Listen to the sounds of the woods, a bell tolling in the distance, tea being poured into your cup, your cat's

AR

purr. Hearing is not bound by only the five senses. Intuition is the sixth sense and should not be forgotten. Rely on it. Take a new path, stop and listen to a piece of music, draw a card from a tarot deck and let it speak to you. Listen to your feelings. How are you right now? What do you feel you need? What can you let go of? Breathe, center yourself, and simply be present with all your senses.

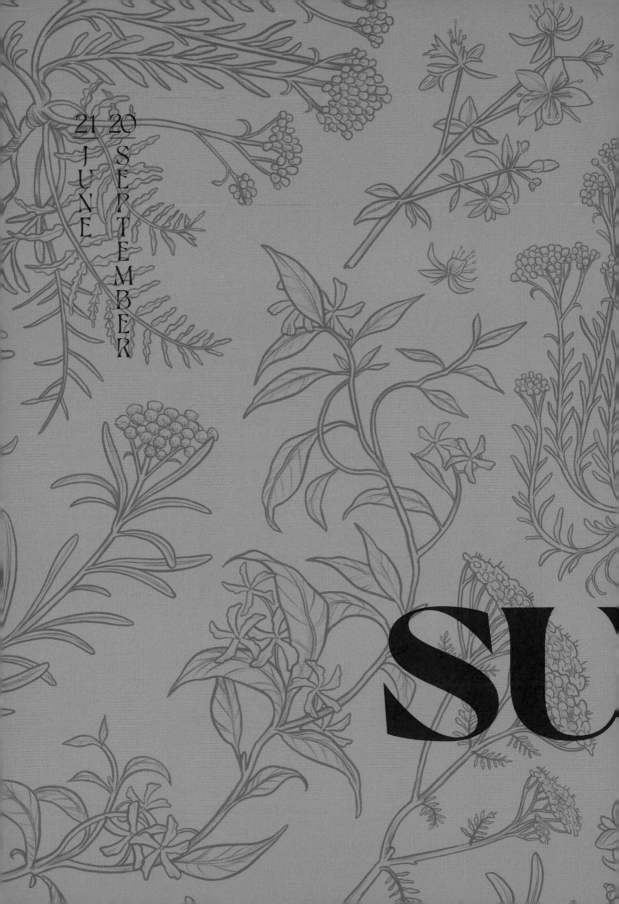

21 JUNE

20 SEPTEMBER

SU

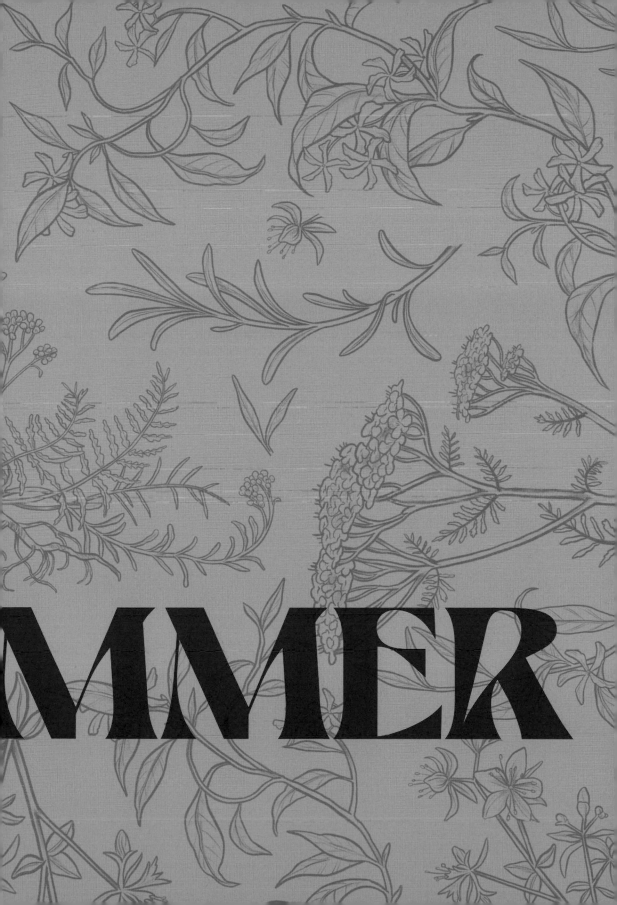

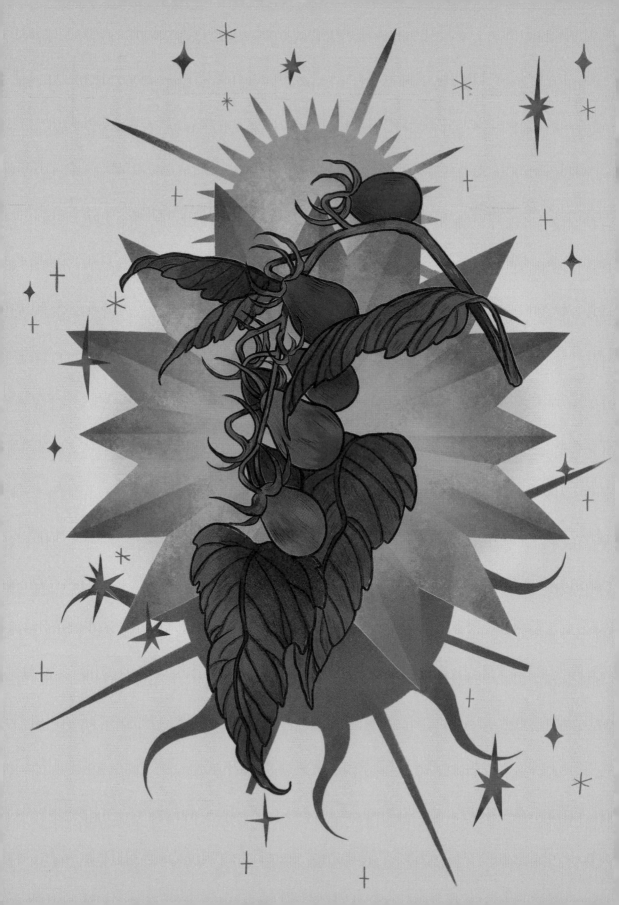

FRUIT

This is a time of wonder, the time to gather the fruits.

Wake up in the summer; step outside, and realize it is time to harvest apricots, perfectly ripe and warm, the color of the sun. Enter the garden and greet the tomatoes, which have slowly changed from green to red.
Light floods our time in this season. Around the summer solstice, the days stretch out in a kaleidoscope of pink, orange, violet, and indigo, before fading into warm evenings lit by fireflies and accompanied by cricket song. The season itself becomes fruit, to be picked and wholeheartedly savored. Let the sweet juice quench your thirst just like a slice of mango enjoyed as you sit by the sea, watching the shooting stars and making wishes. Fruit is a symbol of fullness, completed work, abundance, and fulfillment. It holds the seeds of desires and plans for the future that will come to life in the new spring.

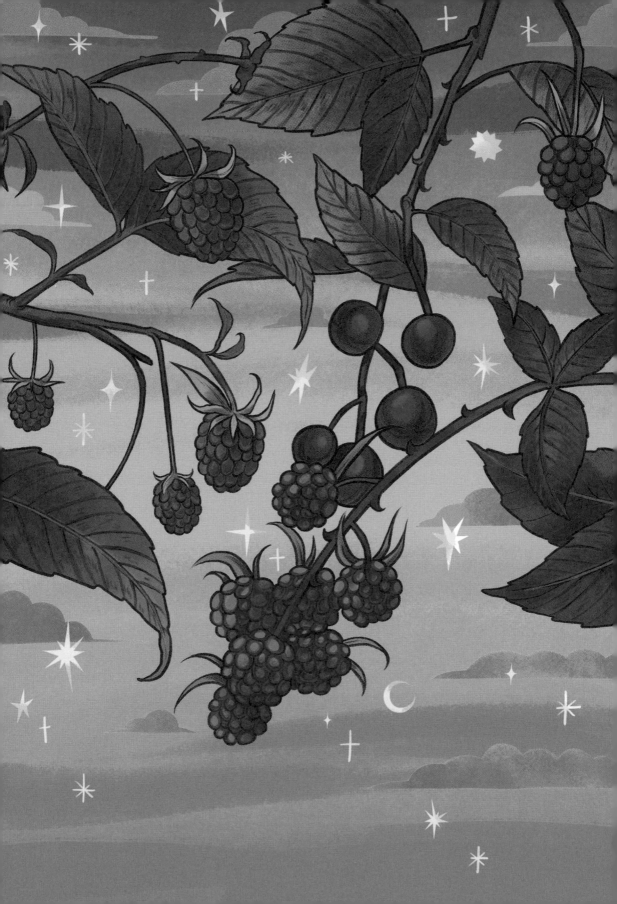

THE FOREST IN SUMMER

In the forest, you can discover summer by observing the light and colors.

Entering the forest means finding shade and refreshment under a large oak tree or among the roots of a chestnut tree. The forest welcomes those who wish to walk, to finally read that book, or to simply rest in the kind shade. You'll know that summer has arrived when it only takes a few steps into the woods to find a blackberry or raspberry bush. Put a berry in your mouth and let it melt to savor the fullness of the season. Entering the beech forest in summer means plunging into the emerald green of June. The scent in the air is different; both the forest and the herbana witch can smell it. St. John's Wort (*Hypericum perforatum*) begins to bloom on the side of the trail, and its intense scent mingles with that of the laurel blossoms (*Prunus laurocerasus*), which smell of almonds and cookies. In the evening, when the herbana witch strains her ears, she hears the wild boars approaching outside her house to eat the apples she left for them or to munch on some acacia (*Robinia pseudoacacia*) flowers.

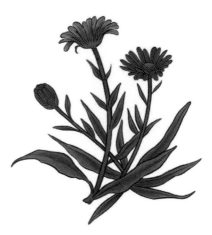

In summer, we experience the triumph of light. The summer solstice, which falls around June 21, is the longest day of the year. From this time on, the days will gradually, imperceptibly shorten until we reach the autumnal equinox, when light and darkness balance each other out. During the summer season, we experience brightness, radiance, and communication. We spend more time outside of the house during this season, so it's the right time to change your perspective by making new friends, familiarizing yourself with new habits and places, and having fun.

This season can be difficult for those who are more introverted. If you, like the herbana witch, need space and solitude to recharge your batteries, remember that along with the light, summer also brings darkness. The summer night is filled with stars and wishes, granting us the chance to laze around and enjoy the beauty that surrounds us.

Summer is the time of fruit and thus fulfillment. You can reflect on what you sowed during the spring— new projects, fresh relationships, or changes in any other area of your life— and observe how these changes have developed.

Get deeply in touch with your body in this season. Feel how alive and vibrant it is, and welcome your body exactly as it is right now.

Explore your day with all your senses. In summer, seek out the presence of water, an important element. Spend time near the water, whether it be a river, a lake, or the sea; get in touch with the fluidity and freshness of the element, with its depth and strength.

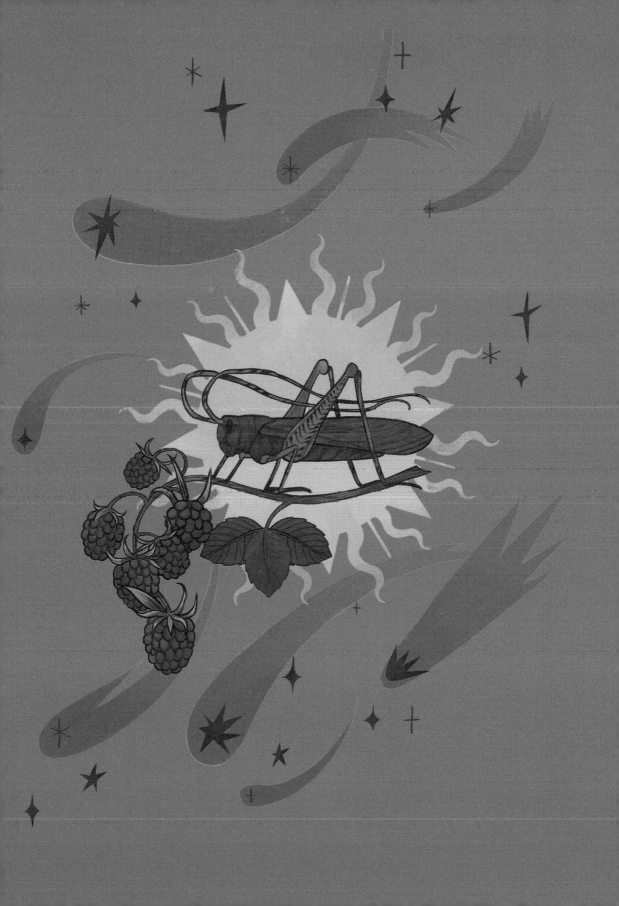

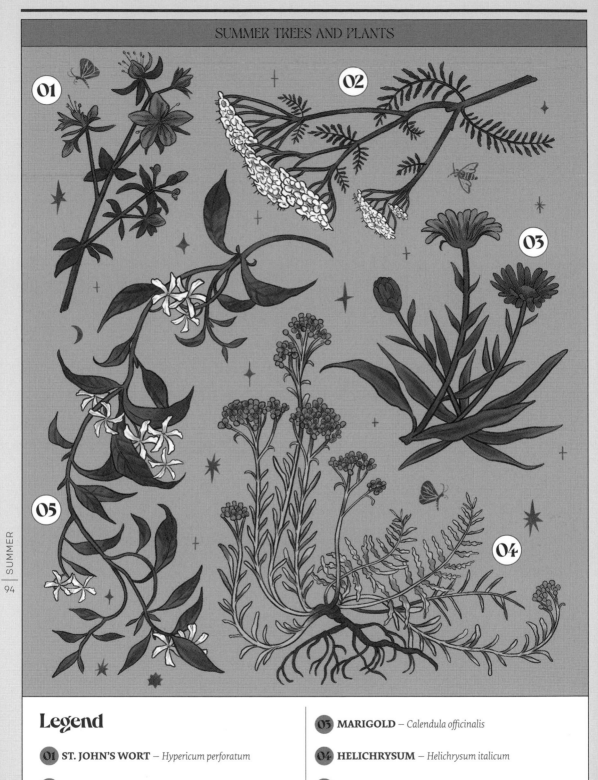

Legend

01 **ST. JOHN'S WORT** — *Hypericum perforatum*

02 **YARROW** — *Achillea millefolium*

03 **MARIGOLD** — *Calendula officinalis*

04 **HELICHRYSUM** — *Helichrysum italicum*

05 **JASMINE** — *Jasminum officinale*

Summer Trees and Plants

This is the season of sunshine. Summer plants and trees have warm colors, ranging from yellow to red, and are rich and tasty plants. Very often they come to our aid with properties that help treat rashes, sunburn, irritation, and heat stroke. The power of the sun can also be used to prepare macerated oils by steeping herbs in oil and exposing them to the sun's rays.

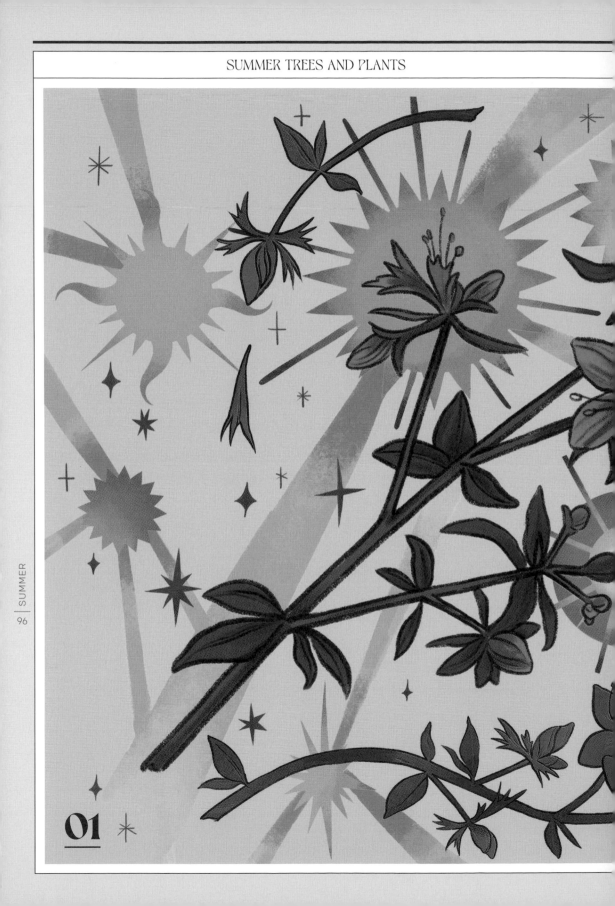

01

St. John's Wort

St. John's wort blooms in the days around the summer solstice, between June 21 and 24, and so takes its name from the feast day of St. John the Baptist. St. John's wort is a solar plant. It absorbs summer heat and brightness to later release them in the colder months through concoctions that help soothe, warm, and relax muscle tension. It is a plant that brightens and brings light. Its property is not only external but also internal. This almost dim-looking seedling shines along the forest edge and seems to say that darkness will pass if we trust in the light. In phytotherapy, St. John's wort is used as an antidepressant. Its active ingredients, hypericin and hyperforin, affect the reuptake of serotonin, a chemical linked to positive mood. St. John's wort can improve your mood and bring light back to even the saddest soul. However, it can interact with many medications; consult a physician to make sure it isn't contraindicated. Preparing a macerated oil by steeping freshly picked flowers in olive oil and exposing them to the sun for about a month is one of the herbana witch's favorite celebrations of summer.

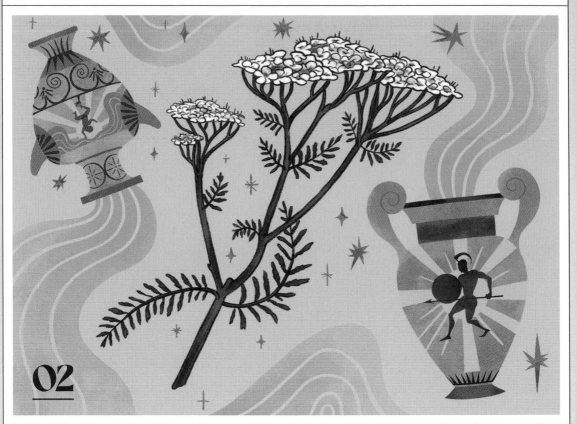

02

Yarrow

Yarrow is one of the unmistakable signs that summer has arrived in the woods. It begins blooming in June and continues until the end of August, accompanying evening walks and nature explorations with its aromatic scent. At first glance, it looks like a slender, delicate flower. To know its strength you must caress it. Feel its stem, which is strong, stiff, rooted, and stretches toward the sky. Yarrow, or *Achillea millefolium*, is named after the invincible warrior Achilles, who was protected, it is said, by a bath infused with the plant when he was a child. It is one of the most suitable plants for healing wounds, both physical and spiritual. When blended with mint, it can heal the wounds of the heart. When the macerated oil is applied to the skin, it is healing and soothing, and it improves capillary fragility. Yarrow was once used for divination; an ancient I-Ching method involved throwing yarrows sprigs in order to read the future. The herbana witch always keeps a jar of yarrow to heal the wounds of a broken heart, or to burn a few leaves on charcoal as incense.

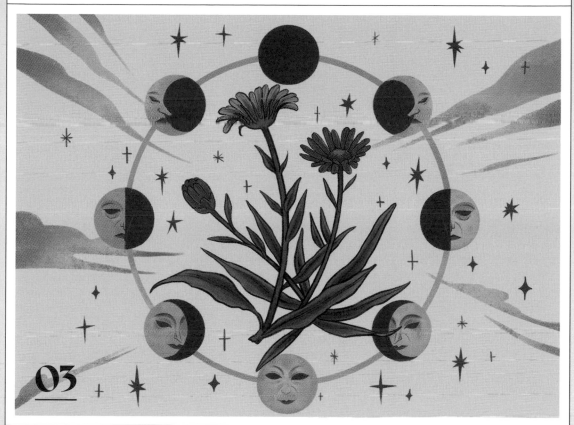

03

Marigold

Marigold and its sappy scent tell of a different kind of fire than other summer plants. The warmth of this plant is related to everything that is intimate, internal, feminine, and cyclical. Its name, *Calendula officinalis*, comes from the ancient Roman lunar calendar, in which the *calenda* marked the monthly rising of the moon. The marigold seed is sickle-shaped, just like the crescent moon, and its flowering lasts a lunar cycle. It can bloom every month in mild weather conditions. It is precisely because of these characteristics that the herbana witch uses marigold wisely, whenever a soft, gentle warmth is required. Use marigold to treat rashes, redness, and minor burns; in the winter, use it for frostbite or cracked skin. Taken internally, it regulates the menstrual cycle and cleanses the liver, intestines, and kidneys. To make an herbal marigold tea, pick its orange flower heads and set them out to dry. They add color and release their beneficial properties to teas and infusions.

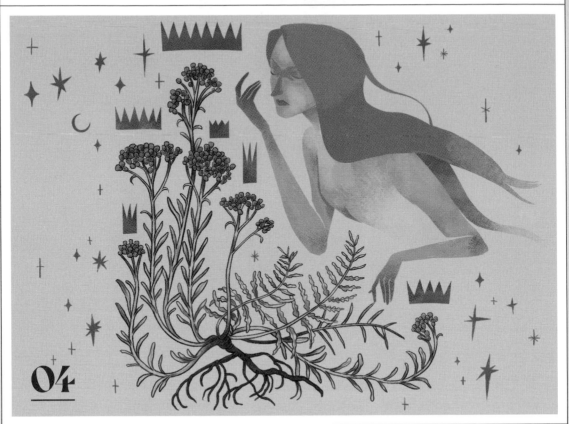

04

Helichrysum

When we find helichrysum, we are in the presence of the queen of summer. Its appearance reveals everything about this season, from its silvery leaves to its ever-blooming golden yellow flowers to its unmistakable scent of licorice and salt. Helichrysum has a powerful cleansing effect, much like what happens when we leave for vacation at the height of summer. We take only the essentials, leaving all our unnecessary baggage at home. Helichrysum is a purifier for the liver and allergies. It should be ingested with caution. Helichrysum has a strong detoxifying effect which can quickly push accumulated toxins out of the body through the skin. As a macerated oil, it is very useful for psoriasis, a common treatment in herbal medicine. In the case of eye allergies, the herbana witch prepares a warm infusion to be applied to the area to calm the itching and counter the allergic reaction.

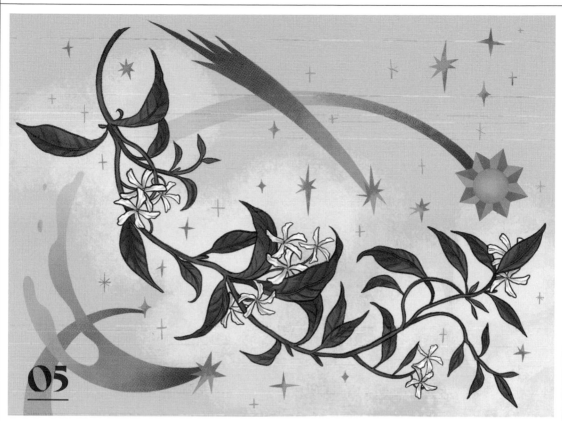

05

Jasmine

The scent of jasmine seems to come from the fireflies and summer stars. Its scent is both unmistakable and mellow, a symbolic fragrance of the season known for its ability to open one up to love and pleasure. According to an Arab legend, jasmine flowers are stars that have fallen to earth. Connected to the summer moon, jasmine is an expression of the feminine and possesses Venusesque and sensual elements. It is a plant that affects both the psycho-emotional and sexual spheres. Jasmine essential oil is one of the most valuable in the world—a true magical spirit. Its calming scent relieves tension, anxiety, and restlessness, and also bestows strength and vitality. Its dual nature is also found in the plant's appearance: the flowers, white and delicate, bloom on a strong and vigorous plant. Massages with its essential oil, diluted in almond oil, on the belly can stimulate regular and full menstruation, and, because it is used as a uterine tonic, it can be used in lumbar massages during childbirth. It has strong aphrodisiac powers and awakens all the senses.

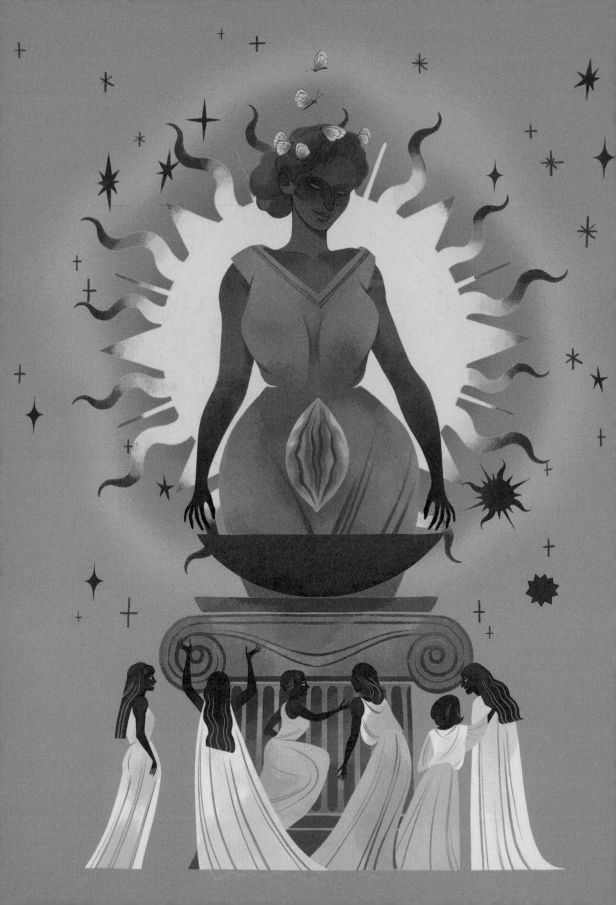

HONEY BREAD

In summer, the herbana witch makes a special bread with ancient roots. It is kneaded with sesame seeds and honey, an ingredient that seems to come straight from the sun.

Luciana Percovich, in her book *Oscure Madri Splendenti*, talks about melloi, sweet breads with a peculiar vulvar shape, dedicated to the goddess Demeter. These loaves, whose shape hints at the creation of life—symbolizing fertility, nourishment, and feminine power—were kneaded with flour, honey, and sesame seeds, ingredients equally rich in meaning. Honey is produced by bees, sacred animals symbolizing abundance and industriousness, whereas sesame seeds symbolize death and rebirth. In India, in ancient times, four pots of black sesame were offered in funeral rites; at the same time, sesame is a symbol of life and fertility, thanks to the great variety of its seeds and the bountiful production of them by plants.

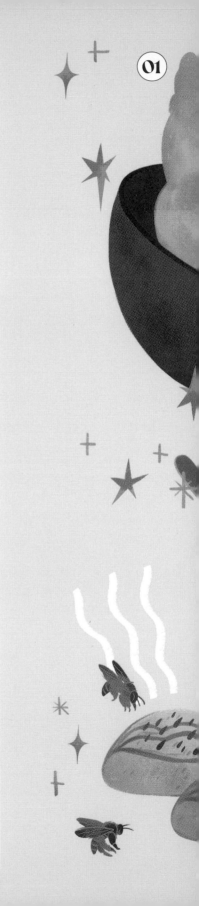

SECRET RECIPE

Dissolve the yeast or sourdough starter in warm water, in a fairly large bowl **01**. Add flour slowly, working it into the water and kneading well **02**. Add the honey and continue kneading until you get a soft, smooth dough **03**. Cover with a clean cloth and let rise in a sheltered place for at least 3–4 hours **04**. Afterward, divide the dough into several balls. Knead again briefly and shape them before leaving them to rise for another hour **05**. Before baking, lightly moisten the surface of the bread with water and sprinkle with sesame seeds **06**. Bake in the oven at 350°F (180°C) for about half an hour.

INGREDIENTS

→ **8 CUPS (1 KG) FLOUR**
→ **1¼ CUPS (300 G) SOURDOUGH STARTER
   OR 2.5 TABLESPOONS BAKER'S YEAST**
→ **5 TABLESPOONS (100 G) HONEY**
→ **3 TABLESPOONS OLIVE OIL**
→ **SESAME SEEDS**
→ **A PINCH OF SALT**
→ **LUKEWARM WATER, AS MUCH AS IS NEEDED**

HONEY

Honey has been considered a sacred food since ancient times because it can both preserve and nourish, and because it is produced by bees, a divine symbol of regeneration, life, and abundance. A true superfood, honey comes from the nectar of flowers, which is processed by bees. Honey is energetic, rich in vitamins and minerals, and has many beneficial properties. It contains a large percentage of fructose, a simple sugar, and has strong antiseptic, anti-inflammatory, and decongestant characteristics. Because it is produced by the nectar from different plants, it can be enriched by the specific characteristics of those plants. Eucalyptus honey, for example, has soothing properties just like the plant. A spoonful of honey dissolved in an herbal tea can heal you, warm you, and make you feel at home.

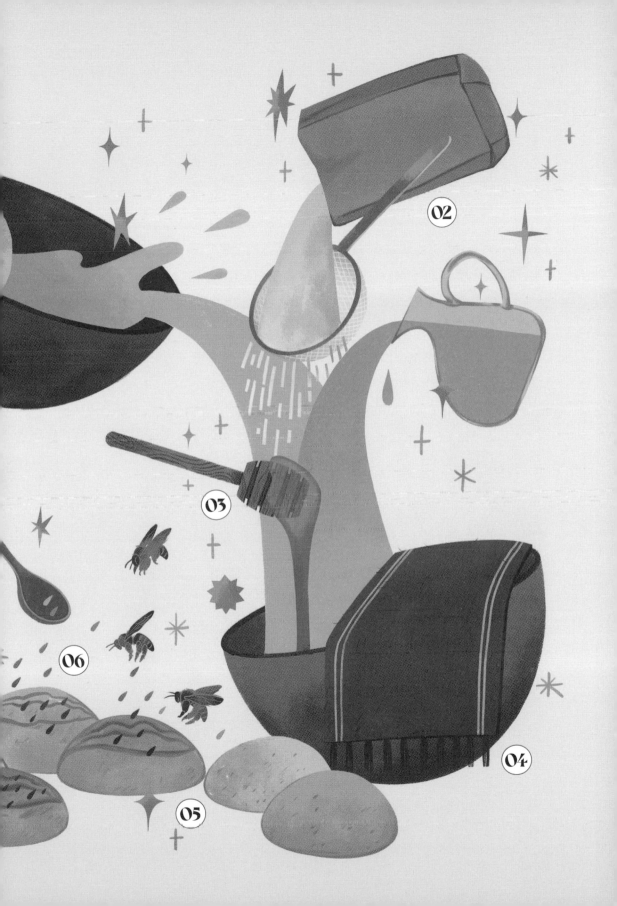

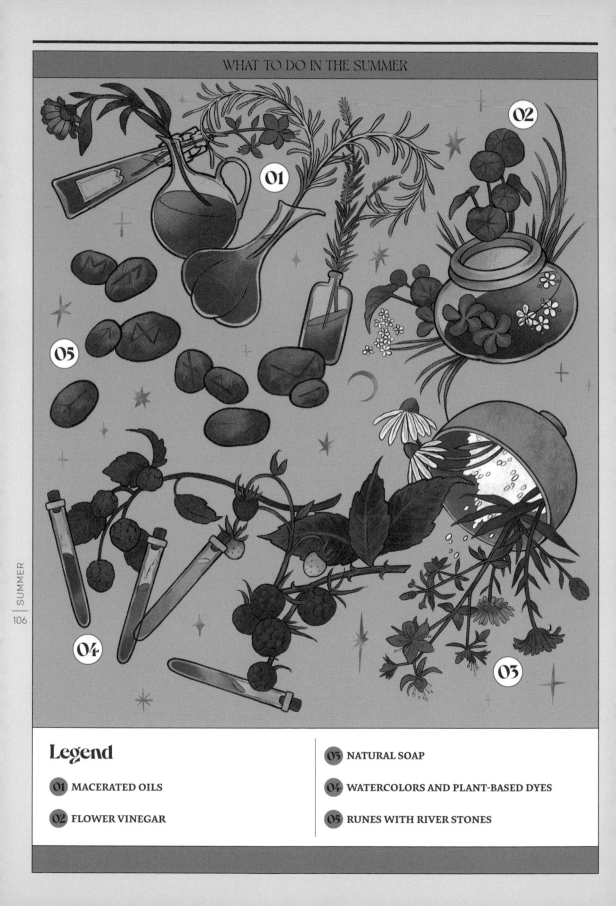

Legend

01 **MACERATED OILS**

02 **FLOWER VINEGAR**

03 **NATURAL SOAP**

04 **WATERCOLORS AND PLANT-BASED DYES**

05 **RUNES WITH RIVER STONES**

What to Do in the Summer

For the herbana witch, summer is about harvesting, preparing, and self-care. You only need to go out into the woods to find beneficial plants and exquisite fruits that can be made into fragrant oils or natural soaps. Nature is so rich and lush that it makes you want to paint it. Extracting color from the plants can allow you to create small magical pieces, infused with the vital energy of the fruits. This is the most suitable time to gather and transform herbs, to take care of your beauty and your soul, and to listen to the teachings of the fireflies. The plants of summer can be used for the preparations you find here, especially macerated oils.

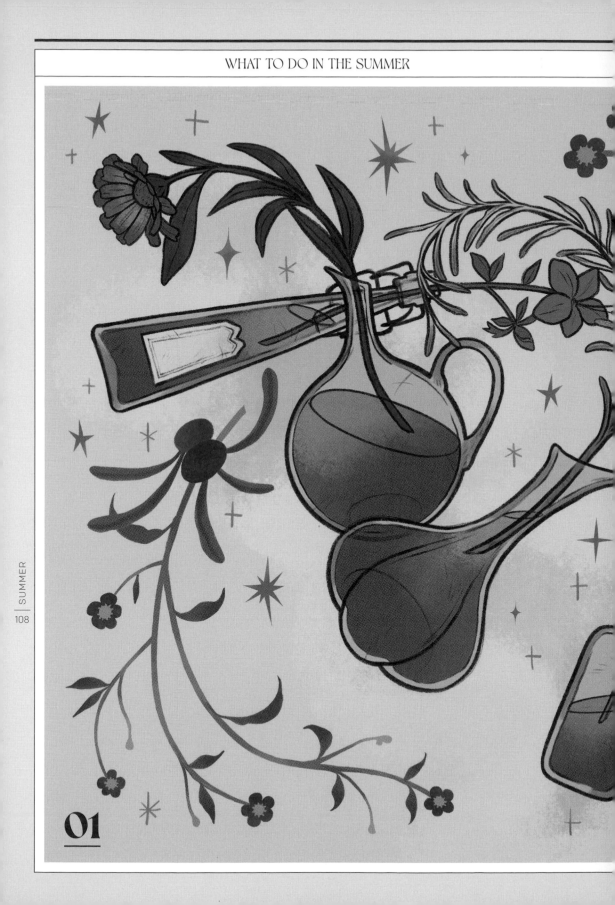

01

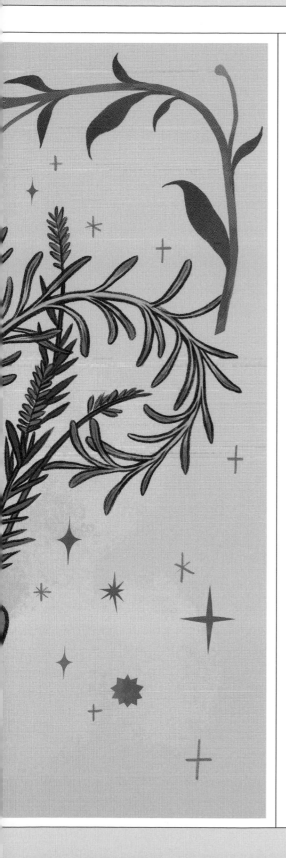

Macerated Oils

Summer is the best time to create macerated oils, which are made by steeping the fresh plant in vegetable oil. These oils are intended for external use. During the maceration process, the plant releases fat-soluble substances into the oil. This makes the preparation both fragrant and useful, enriching the oil with the plant's beneficial properties. To make your own macerated oils, collect the fresh plant (St. John's wort, marigold, lavender, helichrysum, etc.) and place it in a glass jar. Cover the plant with cold-pressed olive or sunflower oil, secure the top of the jar with gauze held in place by a rubber band, and place in the sun for four weeks. Strain and store in dark-colored glass bottles. Before choosing what kind of macerated oil to make, check which plants have which properties and select a plant best suited for your purposes.

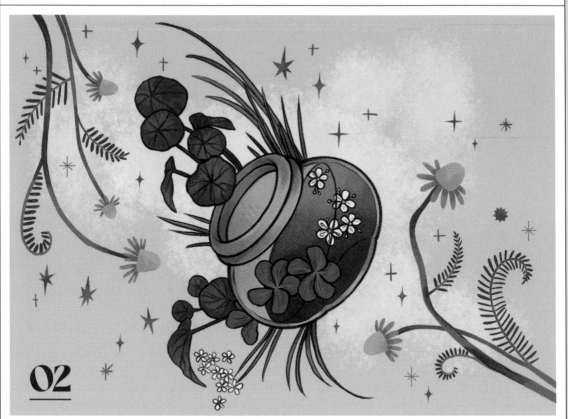

02

Flower Vinegar

Season your summer salads by infusing vinegar with flowers and fruits. You can use elderflower, lavender, nasturtium, chives, or mint, as well as some dried or fresh spices such as garlic, cinnamon, cloves, or ginger. Place about 7 ounces (50 g) of flowers and spices in an airtight jar and cover them with 2 cups (0.5 l) of apple cider or wine vinegar. Let it steep for five days in a cool, shady place. Strain and use to season your summer vegetables! If you prefer fruit, cover 7 ounces (200 g) of fresh fruit (raspberries, blueberries, currants) with 2 cups (0.5 l) of vinegar and seal tightly. Let sit for two weeks in a cool, shady place, then strain and use as you like. You can use any kind of vinegar: wine vinegar, apple cider vinegar, or even a kombucha vinegar. Just remember to use unpasteurized vinegar so that the vinegar's natural probiotic properties remain intact.

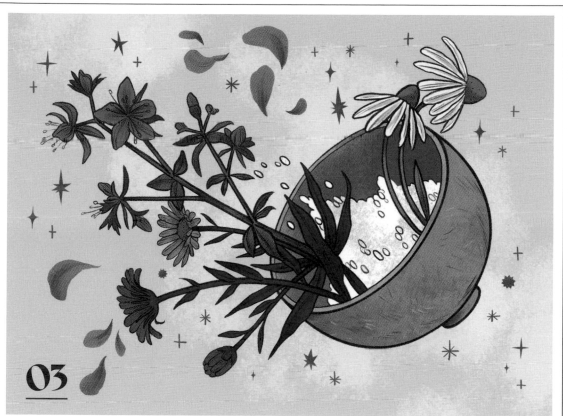

03

Natural Soap

Make new soaps using herbs and flowers from the summer woods. These soaps are wonderful to hang by the shower or take camping. This simple activity is great to do with children. Take 9 ounces (250 g) of Marseille soap and grate it finely. Put it in a bowl and combine summer flower petals, such as poppy, calendula, chamomile, mint, lavender, helichrysum, and rose, and a few tablespoons of almond oil. If you want, you can add a few drops of the essential oil of your choice at this time to intensify the scent. Knead until you get a smooth consistency. With slightly damp fingers, take the soap paste and form spheres. Let them dry on a sheet of baking paper in a cool, dry place. Now you have soap to enjoy!

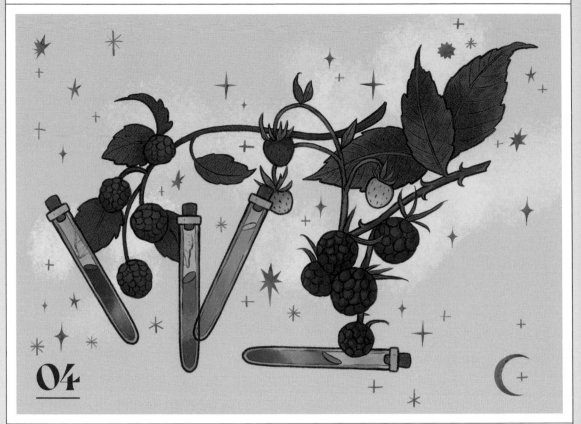

04

Watercolors and Plant-Based Dyes

You can create real plant-based watercolors from summer fruits and flowers. Blueberries, elderberries, blackberries, and raspberries will become shades ranging from red to purple; nettle leaves and spinach make a delicate green; strawberries for red; and tea leaves or coffee for warm brown tones. You'll need to choose the fruits and plants, sort them by color, and then squeeze out the juice. To do this, put them in a clean cotton cloth and wring it out tightly over a funnel inside a bowl. Use the colorful juice collected as a watercolor with suitable brushes and paper. Plant-based colors tend to change over time if exposed to sunlight, so protect your work when finished. To create special patterns and designs, paint the back of leaves with clear veins and then stamp them on watercolor paper. This will give you delicate and striking designs.

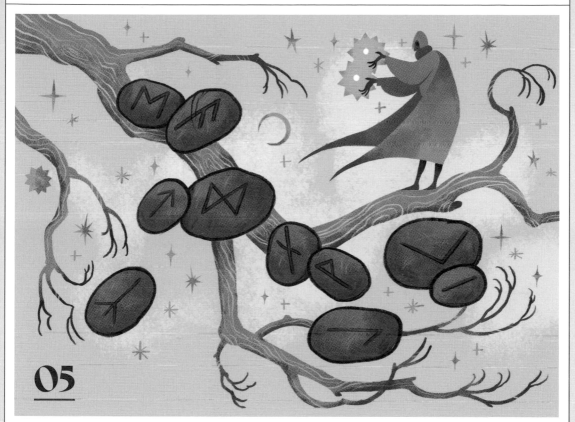

05

Runes with River Stones

Water is linked to divination because of its of fluidity and depth. To get more in touch with this element and its power, you can make your own set of runes by collecting river stones. Runes are an ancient magical alphabet, said to have been given to Odin after his sacrifice at the tree of life, Yggdrasill, from which he hung for seven days and seven nights. At the end of this time, he was deprived of human sight but received the runic alphabet, thus great magical and divinatory power. Carefully choose twenty-four stones, one for each letter of the runic alphabet. The stones shouldn't be too large or too small, and should fit comfortably in the palm of your hand. Paint each stone with a runic symbol until you have the entire alphabet. Consecrate this process close to water. Now you are ready to use your own personal runes.

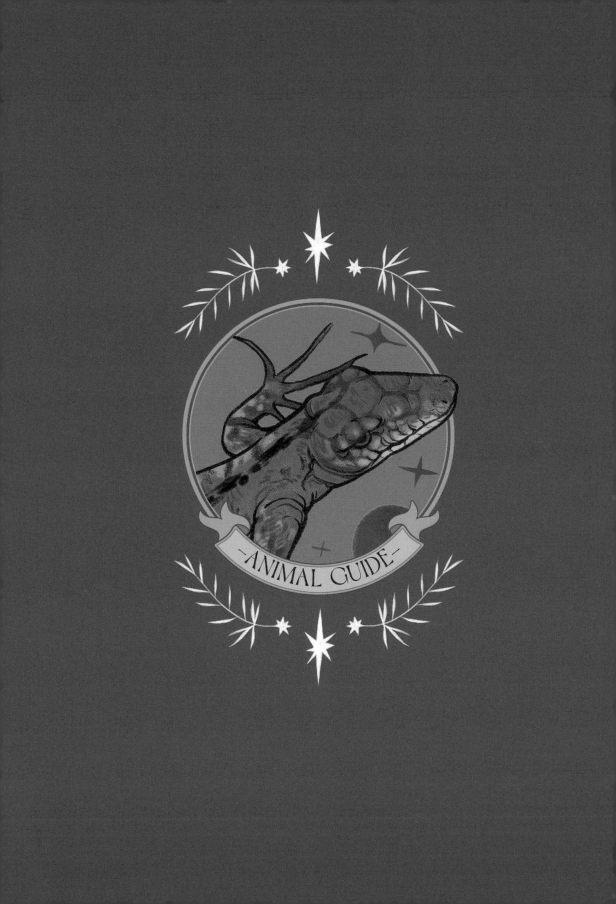

-ANIMAL GUIDE-

THE LIZARD

The lizard seems
almost lifeless, motionless
in the August sun.
But all it takes is a little
noise to startle it.

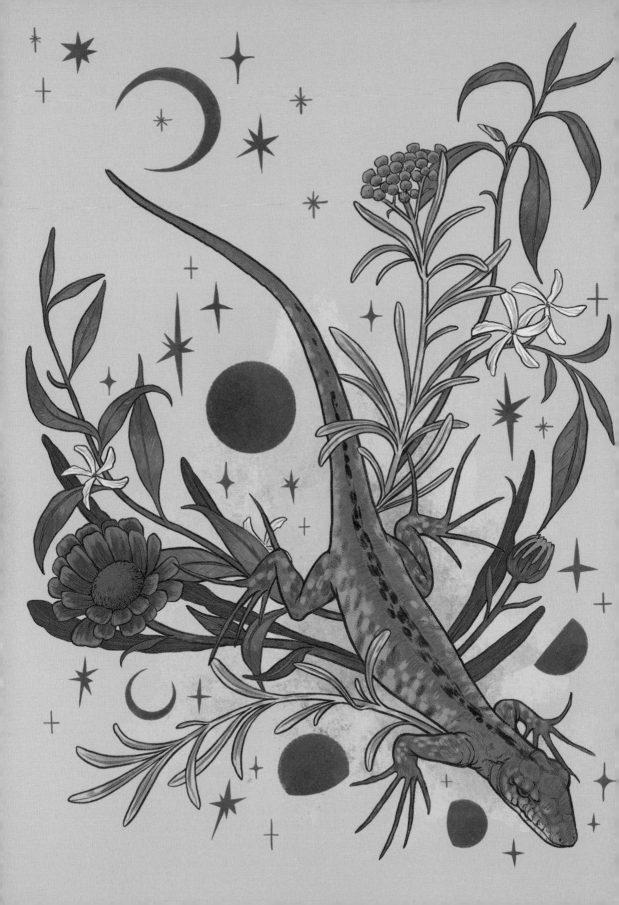

The lizard is associated with the ability to survive, and also with dreaming. **This magical animal** *gifted a stage name to* **Jim Morrison***, lead singer of one of the most psychedelic bands ever, The Doors, who in* **Celebration of the Lizard** *declared* **"I'm the Lizard King, I can do anything."**

A SYMBOL OF transformation, death, and rebirth, the lizard is closely related to the sun because of its characteristic of emerging from small, shadowy cracks into the light and warmth.

Its unique ability to remain still makes it symbolic of observation. The lizard sheds its skin several times during its life cycle and, if its tail is severed, the lizard manages to not only survive, but regenerate the missing body part. This renders the lizard a symbol of strength, mystery, and the capacity for vital regeneration.

The lizard is a shamanic and sacred animal. The ancient Greeks associated it with Apollo, the sun god. The lizard is present as a symbol on many funerary monuments from the classical era, as it was associated with immortality. Its symbolic characteristics also hark back to the myth of Hades and Persephone.

Persephone was destined to live for six months in the underworld and six months above the Earth, bringing with her the light and rebirth of spring and summer.

In Native American mythology, the lizard is an animal of dreams, the one who uncovers light and hidden meanings. It is animal-medicine, representing the hidden dark side without which the bright side cannot shine.

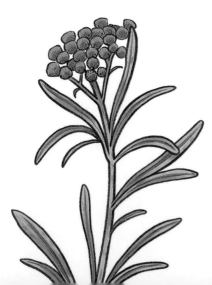

NURT

THE HERBANA WITCH'S MESSAGE

In summer, more than any other season, recharge yourself with sunshine, freshly harvested fruits, rest, and activities that connect you with the natural world. Sunbeams hitting the windowsill invite you to do as the lizard does; ripe tomatoes, in the garden or on the balcony, are delicious and barely warm; running your fingers across basil leaves nourishes your thoughts and brings beauty and magic. Where do you get your nourishment from? What really satiates you? What brings you satisfaction? To receive nourishment, you have to know where to look for it. In summer,

TURE

work on your ability to ask for exactly what you want. But remember, says the herbana witch, that you might actually get it. So exercise willpower and precision, and learn how to receive things wholeheartedly, filling yourself with sunshine and radiance. Once you have achieved fulfillment, you can reciprocate the source of nourishment with a small gift: an apple in the woods for the boar that passes by at dusk, a small prism hanging from a chestnut branch that casts rainbows, a nasturtium plant that will host bees to take care of it. Every act of kindness you do prepares you to receive another.

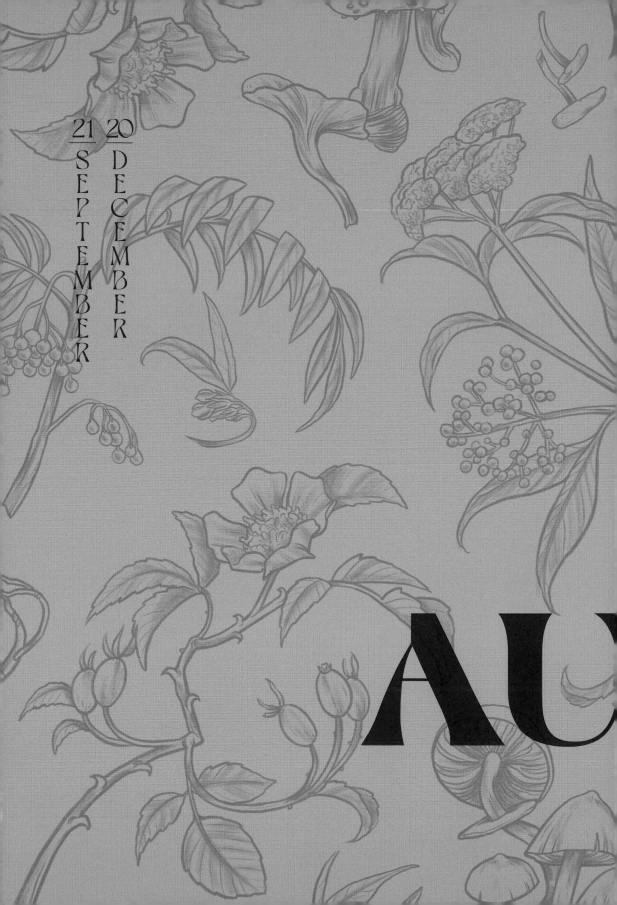

21/SEPTEMBER

20/DECEMBER

AU

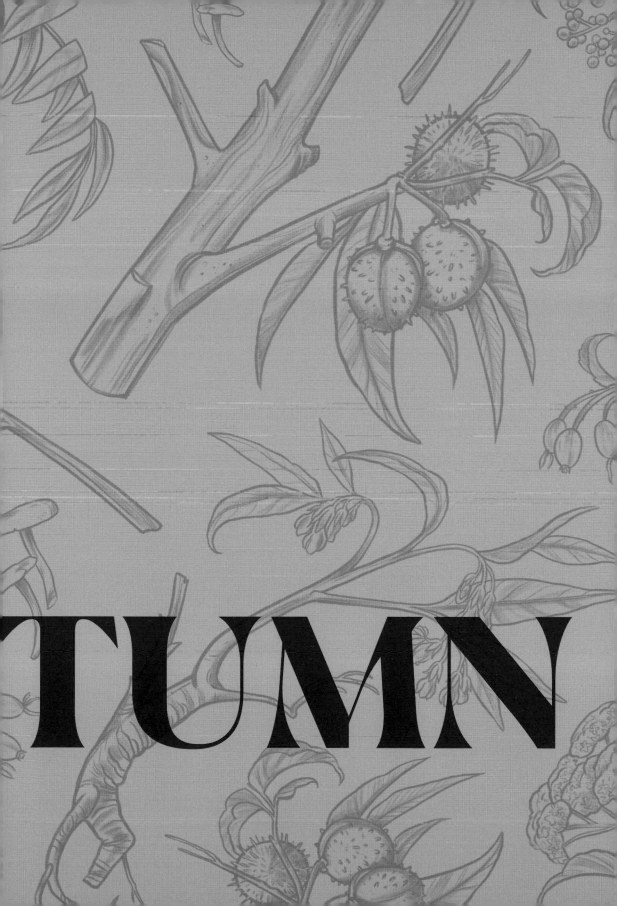

TUMN

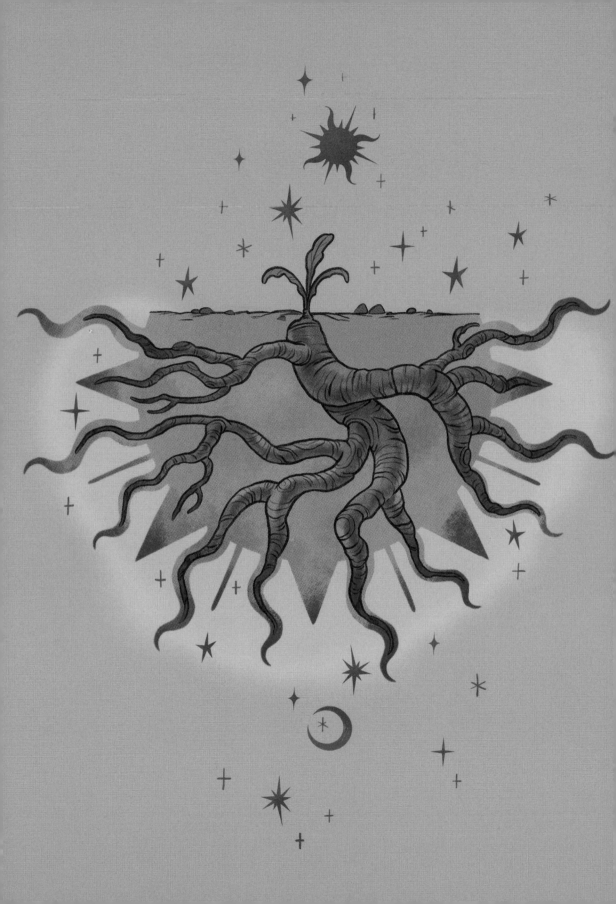

ROOT

In autumn, we slow down, and plants concentrate their energy on the root.

Invisible from the surface, a plant's root grows and expands underground. This is the world of Hades, and this season is when the goddess Persephone returns to the underworld, the subterranean realm that presides over visceral and magical life. This is why roots are often used as amulets. They come from the unknown and are anchored in the earth, so they symbolize vitality, good health, and fertility. The root is the part of the plant that stores nourishment, a reserve for the winter months. Underground, the plant absorbs water, minerals, and nutrients that it will need in the most difficult times. The root is also the means by which plants move. It is a true directional sensory organ, guiding the plant and enabling it to communicate with other plants. The root teaches us to set things aside and seek out what makes us satisfied and safe.

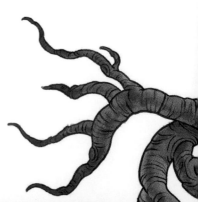

The forest in autumn is a triumph of colors.

On closer inspection, autumn looks like a second spring. The sunshine that the trees received during the summer is given back in the deep red foliage, the orange of sunsets, and the golden yellow of leaves and fruit. Beech forests (*Fagus sylvatica*) are like enchanted worlds. The leaves turn red, and the light that filters through is amber-hued. It touches the heart. In autumn, the woods make you feel at home, like your own little living room. Time moves more slowly, in tune with the rhythm of the plants. It is time to fall. The leaves slowly come off the trees; the plants leave seeds on the dark earth, which will protect them during the winter season. The first rose hip berries begin to appear, red hints in the branches and food for animals. Storms wash over the earth after the summer heat, and everything becomes receptive and listens more deeply.

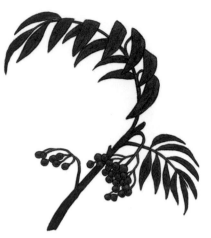

Autumn is harvest time: fruits, small berries, apples, pears, grapes, and olives. There is much work to be done, from harvesting and sorting to transforming and preserving for the colder months. In autumn, movement becomes inward.

While in the spring and summer we are driven to go outside, from autumn on we begin to feel more of a desire for long evenings at home, reading a book or perhaps curled up in front of the fire or under our favorite blanket. A journey into ourselves begins. The equinox, September 21, is a perfect time to take stock of what we have gathered during the year and focus on our goals. This season reminds you that there is a right time for everything. This is the teaching of ivy (*Hedera helix*), with its late blooms.

Ivy flowers in autumn, the last of nectar for bees. Ivy knows its inner rhythm and follows it, resulting in unconventional behavior.

The herbana witch wakes up early in the morning and looks out the small window at the back of her home, the one overlooking the forest. Fog often appears, hazy and soft, reminding us how thin the line is between dreams and reality. Autumn is the season of dreaming. Mushrooms, edible and otherwise, appear in the woods, like the dreaded agarics (*Amanita muscaria*), brightening the fir forests with red and white, the colors of fairy tales. You may encounter them, too, as you follow the red thread of autumn through the woods, from hawthorn berries (*Crataegus oxyacantha*) to maple leaves (*Acer*), like small daytime fireworks against the clear October sky.

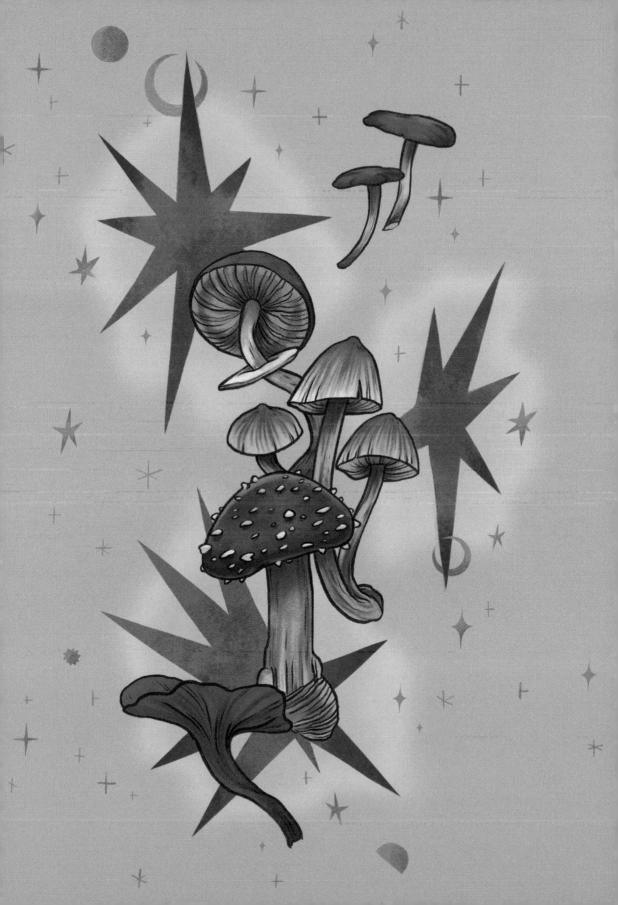

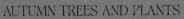

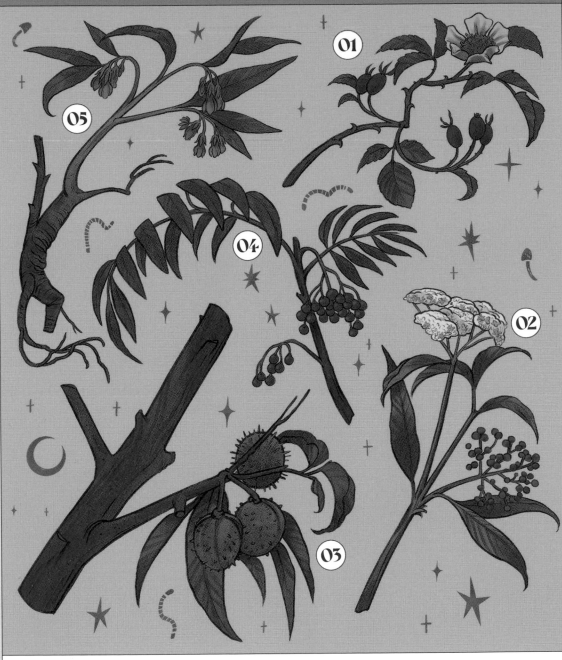

Legend

01 **DOG ROSE** – *Rosa canina*

02 **ELDERBERRY** – *Sambucus*

03 **CHESTNUT** – *Castanea sativa*

04 **SERVICE TREE** – *Sorbus domestica*

05 **COMFREY** – *Symphytum officinale*

Autumn Trees and Plants

In autumn, the plants focus their energy on the root, and the typical berries and stone fruits of the season begin to appear. Autumn is also the time to harvest seeds, such as hazelnuts, almonds, and sunflower seeds. Movement is inward and downward as we enter the most introspective and dreamy season of the year. Fall plants boost immunity, cleanse, and nourish.

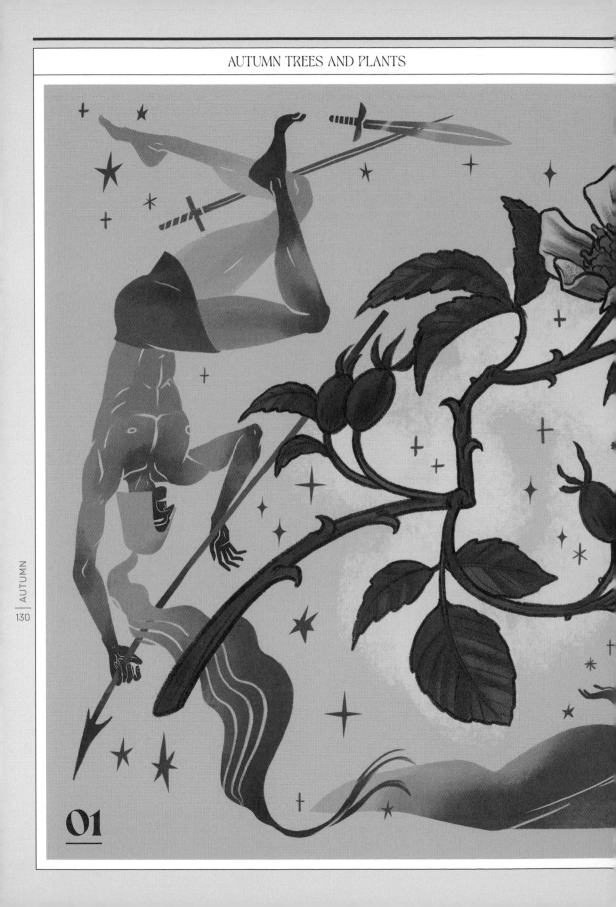

01

Dog Rose

The dog rose is unmistakable, especially in autumn. By October, it becomes highly visible, with its fiery red rose hips popping up on the edges of woods or paths. This plant has a highly developed root system, which gives it great vitality. It is symbolic of both Venus and Mars. We find the former in the delicacy of the flower, the light scent of its petals, and their excellent cosmetic, soothing and moisturizing properties; the latter is evoked by the plant's thorns and the red color of the rose hips, a unique type of berry that is actually a false fruit. Rose hips strengthen the immune system by providing high concentrations of vitamin C, also echoing Mars, a planet that defends and strengthens. It is possible to use rose hips to infuse herbal teas or jams with the color of autumn. After first cutting the rose hips in half, it's important to clean out the seeds as well as the stinging fuzz that surrounds them. The rose hip embraces the duality of flower and thorn, light and darkness, just as nature does on September 21, the day of the autumnal equinox.

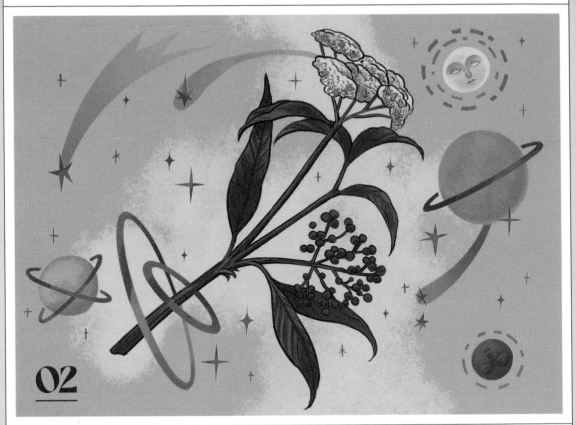

02

Elderberry

A quintessential magical tree connected to the moon and the Wee Folk, elderberry is a threshold tree, living in both this world and the fairy world. Duality is also symbolized in tree's extremities: the full-moon shape within its white flowers, and the black moon within its purple berries. The wood of the elderberry tree, with its symbolic connection to both the moon and Saturn, is perfect for wands. Some parts of the tree are toxic, though a delicious jam can be made from the berries, provided they are ripe and cooked well. If ingested raw, they are harmful. The flowers can regulate body temperature, and are used to treat fevers and colds. They are also used to flavor breads, cakes, and cookies. It is a wise and ancient plant, hence its name. The wand of Albus Dumbledore, a character in J.K. Rowling's Harry Potter series, is made of elder wood, signifying the great wisdom of this powerful wizard.

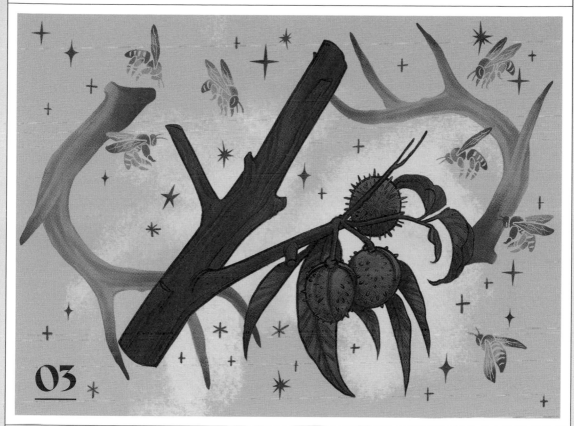

03

Chestnut

The chestnut tree has been cultivated for agriculture since ancient times. It was a means of sustenance in the mountainous regions of Italy and beyond, during times of war and famine. Its fruit is nutritious and hearty and the tree itself is enduring and lush, which is the reason it symbolizes abundance. It is called the "bread tree" because it has fed many people in the mountains with its fruit. Deer, squirrels, and wild boar love chestnuts, and birds find shelter to nest in the tree's branches. Chestnuts are rich in starches and carbohydrates. They can be dried and crushed to produce flour, or boiled/roasted, and added to polenta. Traditionally cradles were made of chestnut wood as symbolic protection for babies. The generosity of this nourishing tree is also found in its relationship with bees. The chestnut tree is called the "bee pantry" because bees collect its nectar to produce chestnut honey. Chestnut honey has an intense color and a slightly bitter taste. It is a real treat.

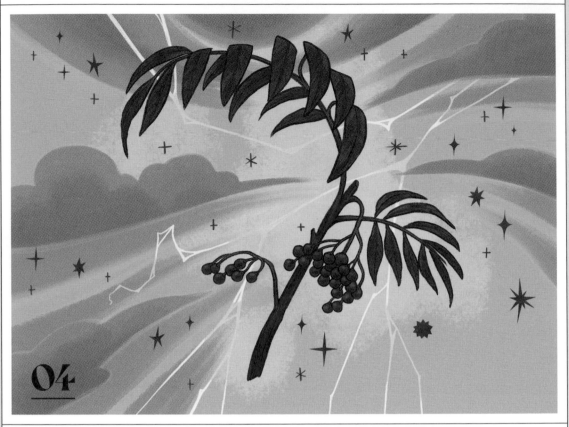

04

Service Tree

The service tree packs all the power of autumn into its small red fruits. These small fruits are called pomes and look like hard berries. They dye the woods red where the tree grows. This tree is an adaptable plant that has been present in domestic gardens since ancient times, said to protect against lightning and bring shelter. Its red color is made manifest in the tree's other name, Rowan, which may come from the Norse raudr, meaning "red." The Irish poet Seamus Heaney described the service tree as "a girl with lipstick." A vital plant, both in bearing and growth, it brings energy through its fruits, which are rich in citric acid and natural sugars. The fruits prevent scurvy and have astringent properties. They make an excellent mouthwash for tonsillitis and sore throats. The service tree is associated with witches. Its branches are suitable both for magic wands and for divining. The service tree is sacred to Brigid, Celtic goddess of fire, passion, and art. Its berries were strung onto red necklaces of protection not only for the inhabitants of a home but also for the animals that lived there.

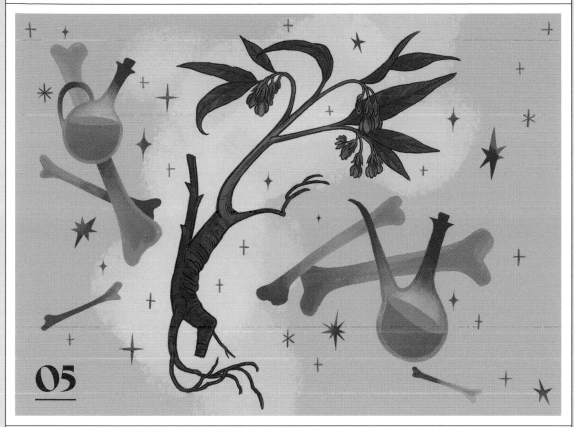

05

Comfrey

Comfrey contains all its magic in its root. It is harvested in late autumn when the leafy green top of the plant has withered. In late summer, the leaves can be harvested. It should be treated with respect and only harvested in places where there are many specimens. The ideal comfrey root is dark on the outside and milky white on the inside. Comfrey has extraordinary healing and restorative abilities. With both the leaves and the root we can make a macerated oil that can be applied whenever there is a need to heal, consolidate, or hold together. The application of comfrey promotes the growth of bone callus, and thus allows for faster repair of fractures. Comfrey is excellent for eczema, mycosis, and rashes; however, it should not be applied to open wounds. Comfrey represents the importance of being together, holding each other, and creating a community.

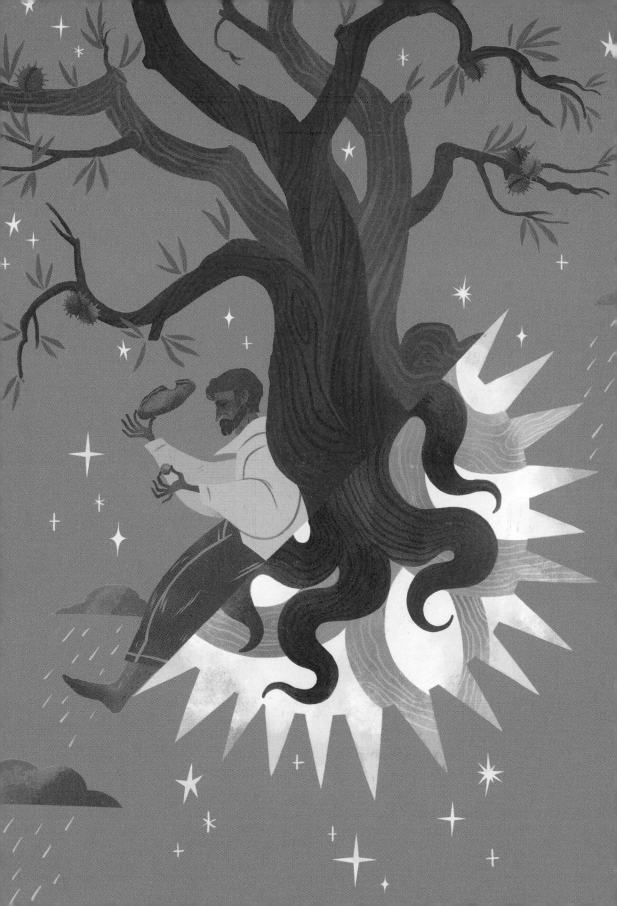

CHESTNUT– FLOUR BREAD

In autumn, make a bread that smells like the forest and mountains, and possesses a sweet and ancient flavor. Bread with chestnut flour is typical of many mountainous regions of Italy, and particularly Tuscany.

In times of war and famine, people in mountainous regions survived on this nutritious fruit, which can also be ground into a flour. Chestnuts were prepared in special structures consisting of small stone buildings with a weave of reeds on which the nuts were placed to dry. A fire was lit underneath and the embers were kept alive for days until the chestnuts were completely dry. After that, they were made into flour! We will make this bread using sourdough as yeast. This is a recommended activity for autumn.

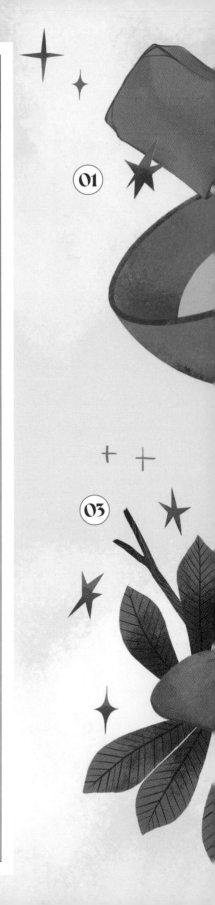

SECRET RECIPE

First, refresh the sourdough starter. The night before making the bread, take your sourdough from the refrigerator, weigh it, and add the same amount of flour and half the amount of warm water **01**. Knead and let it rise until morning. In the morning, take out half a cup (150 g) of this dough and put the remainder in the refrigerator for the next bread-making. Alternatively, you can use dry baker's yeast in the amounts indicated on the packet. Dissolve the sourdough in a bowl with some of the water, then add the bread flour and chestnut flour and knead by adding water until you have a smooth, elastic dough **02**. Knead the bread slowly for at least 10 minutes, enjoying every careful movement as you think about the riches you have and the things that give you nourishment and satisfaction; then let it rise for 4 to 6 hours. After this, knead it lightly, shaping it into whatever shape you prefer. Score the bread with the tip of a knife and wrap it in chestnut leaves if you have them **03**. Let it rise another hour or until doubled in size. Bake at 400°F (200°C) for the first 10 minutes and at 350°F (180°C) for the remaining 30 minutes.

INGREDIENTS

- → 3¼ CUPS (400 G) ALL-PURPOSE FLOUR
- → ¾ CUP (100 G) CHESTNUT FLOUR
- → ½ CUP (150 G) REFRESHED SOURDOUGH STARTER
    OR 2.5 TABLESPOONS BAKER'S YEAST
- → APPROX. 1¼ CUPS (300 ML) WATER

CHESTNUTS

Chestnuts are a very energetic fruit, thanks to the starch and simple sugars they contain. They are rich in folates and B Vitamins, which are beneficial during pregnancy. Chestnuts contain plenty of fiber to help you feel full. They also contain iron, phosphorus, potassium, zinc, magnesium, and calcium. The presence of Vitamin B_6 makes them important in preserving the immune system and metabolism, as well as in regulating hormone production. Chestnuts can be part of many food preparations, both savory and sweet.

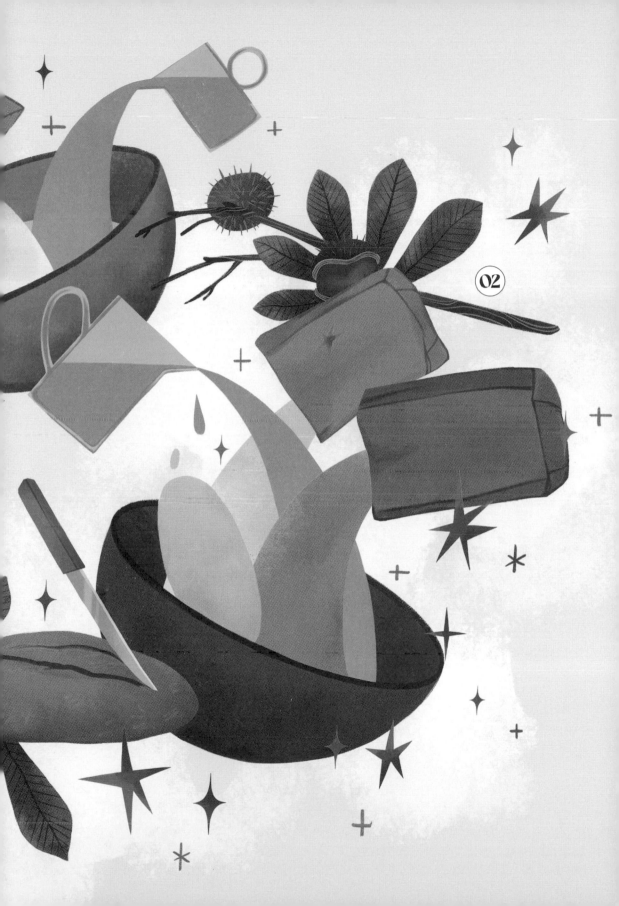

02

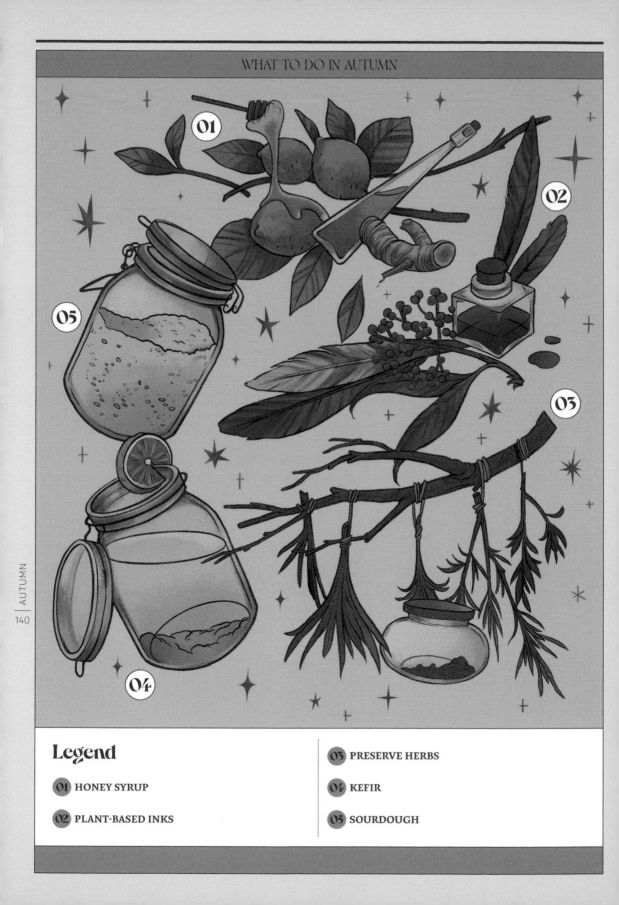

Legend

01 HONEY SYRUP

02 PLANT-BASED INKS

03 PRESERVE HERBS

04 KEFIR

05 SOURDOUGH

What to Do in Autumn

Autumn is a time for gathering, introspection, and observation. The herbana witch prepares for winter, gathers leaves the color of gold, and takes long walks in the woods. She creates a special ink from elderberries with which to write letters on long evenings in front of the fire. In her pantry, sourdough and kefir ferment, alongside herbs that are well preserved in jars. The herbana witch will welcome you to her home with a cup of tea and honey syrup. Use the fall season to slow down, look inward, and take care of your body and home. It is the time of the earth and the root.

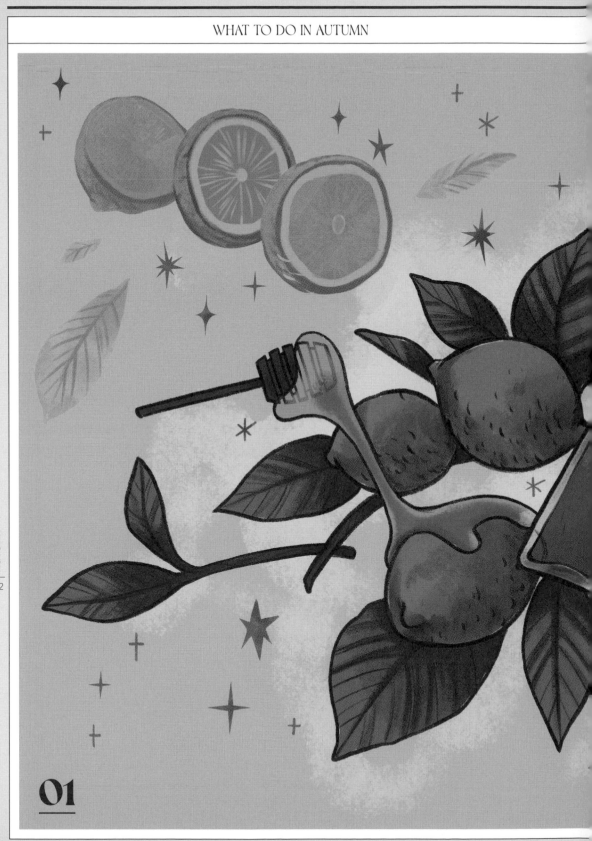

01

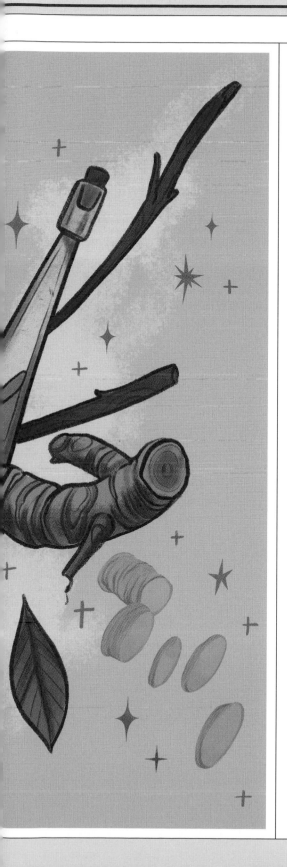

Honey Syrup

In autumn, make a syrup from honey, lemon, and ginger. This syrup is a good, quick remedy for coughs, sore throats, and seasonal ailments. It can also be used to relieve nausea, thanks to the presence of ginger, which has anti-nausea and analgesic properties, and can be effective against headaches, especially if they result from muscle tension or a cold. To prepare the syrup, thinly slice a peeled ginger root and do the same with an organic, untreated lemon (leave the peel on). Put the ginger and lemon in a jar and cover everything with honey, chestnut, eucalyptus, or fir honey. If you use crystallized honey, melt it for a few minutes in a double boiler before pouring. Close the jar and store it in the refrigerator for up to three weeks.

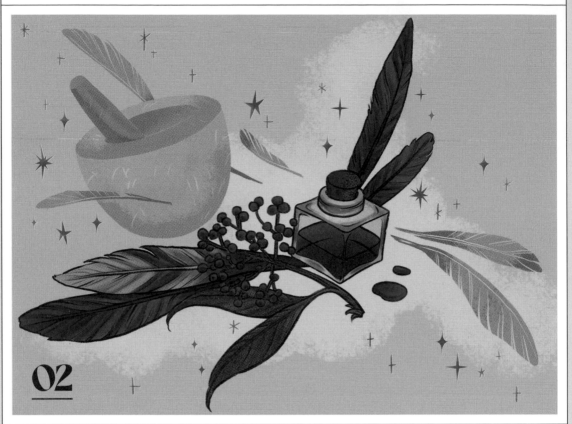

02

Plant-Based Inks

You can make ink with elderberries harvested in late summer. Take a good handful of elderberries, crush them with a fork or in a mortar, and then put them in a pot with twice the volume of water. Boil for about 20 minutes, then strain through a fine-mesh strainer and decant into a glass bottle. To use your elderberry ink, dip a fountain pen, or better yet a feather, into the ink. Elderberry juice contains pigments that release a beautiful purple color, so your writing will be a very elegant dark purple. You can use this ink to write your charms or a special letter, or to jot down your observations about the forest in autumn. You can also dye fabric and even wood using this preparation method. Before dyeing the fabric, remember to treat it with an etchant so that it retains the color.

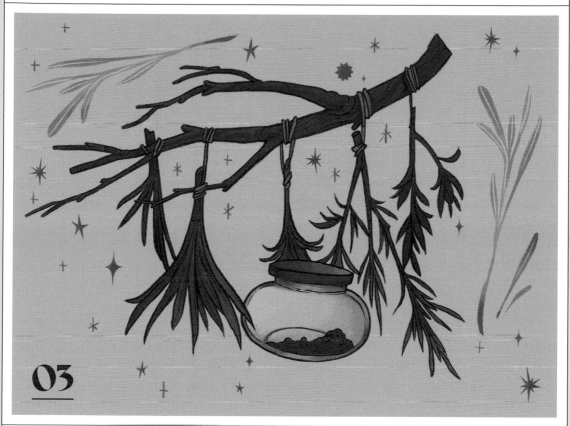

03

Preserve Herbs

The time for harvesting herbs ends in late autumn. By this time they have all been dried, hung upside down in a cool, dry place, and then cut and shredded and placed into glass jars for storage in the pantry. Remember to always put a label on each jar with the name of the plant, the date it was harvested, and, if you like, the phase of the moon in which you harvested it. Keep the jars tightly closed in a place away from light and heat sources. Herbs that have been stored for more than a year should be thrown away. If you can, instead of throwing them in the trash, return them to the earth so that they can fertilize it and potentially scatter seeds that will grow into new seedlings. In the autumn, it is good to tidy up the pantry and herb cupboard, dust, take a small inventory of what you have and what you are missing: collect and transform only what you are sure to use.

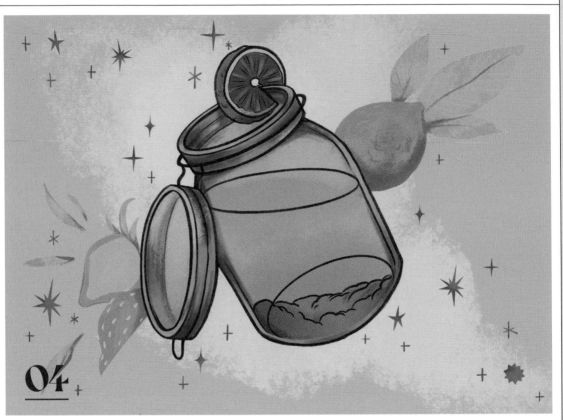

04

Kefir

Both kefir and sourdough are fermented foods with many beneficial properties, helping to replenish intestinal flora while improving and strengthening the immune system. In autumn, it is pleasant to make kefir and knead bread, leaving it to rise in the warmth of the stove. Kefir is a fermented beverage made from agglomerates of lactic-acid bacteria and yeast, called kefir grains. These grains can be "milk" or "water" kefir. Milk kefir grains will ferment animal milk, producing a yogurt-like drink, whereas water kefir grains combined with sugar and lemon will ferment water. Water kefir makes for a fizzy drink! To make water kefir, use 3.5 ounces (100 g) of kefir grains to about 4 cups (1 l) of water, adding 1.5 ounces (40 g) of sugar, two or three dates, and half a lemon. Let it ferment two days, then strain and store in the refrigerator. Rinse the grains and repeat the process.

05

Sourdough

Sourdough is a natural yeast used for making bread. You can make your own sourdough at home with water and flour. Mix about 5 ounces (150 g) of flour with warm water, just enough to produce an elastic dough. Cover with a cloth and leave in a warm place. Every day, for 5 or 6 days, add 3 ounces (90 g) of flour and just enough water. You will see small bubbles begin to form in the dough. This is a sign that it is fermenting! Keep the sourdough in the refrigerator; you will use it in recipes for making bread (always refresh it the night before by adding water and flour and letting it rise). Before baking the bread, take out a small piece of dough and put it in the refrigerator. This will be the sourdough starter, to be used for your next bread-making. A sourdough starter can stay alive many, many years!

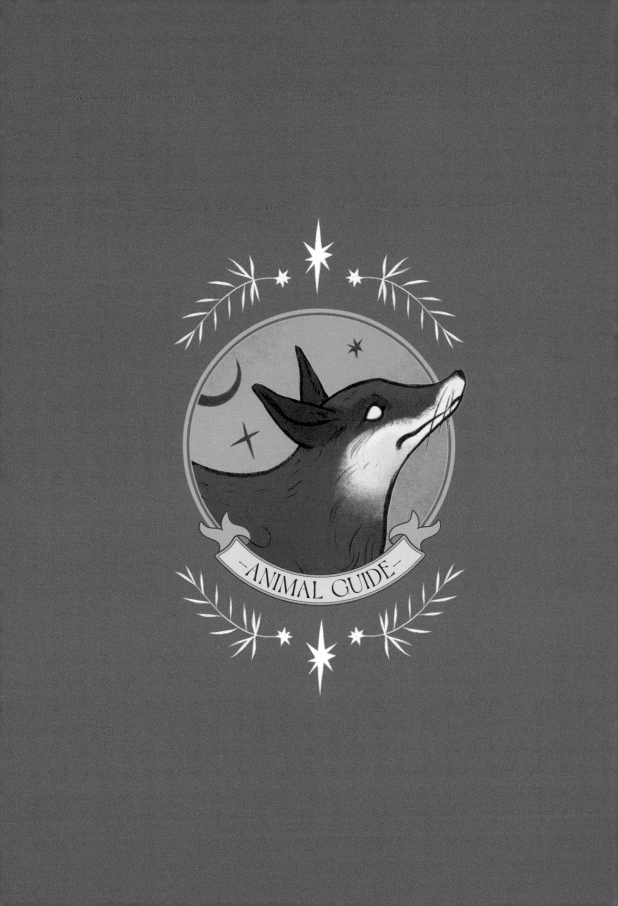

-ANIMAL GUIDE-

THE
FOX

The fox is an animal of
power in many traditions,
often associated
with adaptability
and mutability.

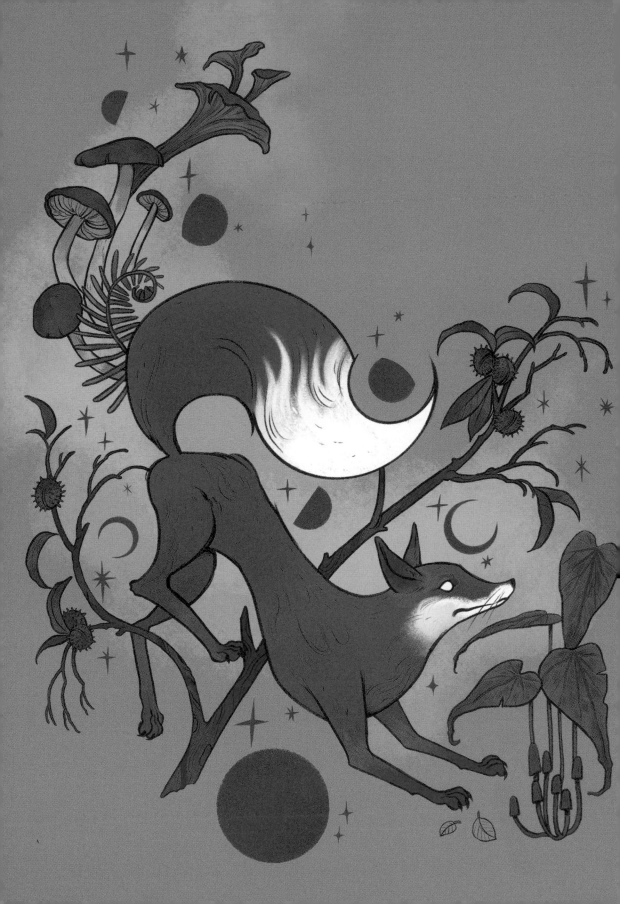

*The fox is just like autumn, a season that changes color and sensations, when nature prepares for winter and slowly transforms. A careful, cautious, and cunning animal, **the fox is a symbol of living intelligence**, the ability to think in alternative ways and find unexpected solutions.*

WALKING IN THE WOODS at dusk, the herbana witch is accompanied by her fox, an orange lightning bolt that goes before her, observes her, and guides her. The Celts considered foxes great connoisseurs of the woods and recognized them as guides, both in the world of the living and the dead.

This animal is associated with the ability to concentrate. When it hunts, it freezes, pointing toward its prey like an arrow. It reminds us that it is necessary to maintain focus, abandoning all distractions.

The famous fox of Antoine de Saint-Exupéry's *The Little Prince* says that "the essential is invisible to the eyes." The connection between foxes and intuitive capacity, linked to subtle and invisible perception, is obvious. Indeed, the fox is close to the world of dreams, ability, and psychic resources: it is a nocturnal animal, although it is also visible during the day.

If you feel akin to the fox in autumn, it could mean that your creative ability is greater at night. According to Japanese folklore, the fox is capable of shape-shifting. This is another sign that connects it to the magical, nocturnal world, which is as ever-changing as the moon. The fox is often associated with tricksters, someone who speaks in riddles, deceives, and performs sly tricks. But the herbana witch knows that the fox is wise and intelligent. He is not dishonest but cunning. He can think clearly, move through the unknown with awareness. The fox suggests that you don't immediately show all your cards, but instead play them strategically. Don't reveal everything; keep it a secret.

COL

THE HERBANA WITCH'S MESSAGE

Collect, and do so with all your senses. Explore the world around you and collect with respect and care. You can collect useless and beautiful things in particular, like a shard of polished glass, an owl feather, a few acorns to make a woodland bracelet. Fall is a good time to stop, slow down, and take stock of what you have collected and what you want. Clean up, tidy up, make preserves for the colder months. Learn something you don't know and would like to

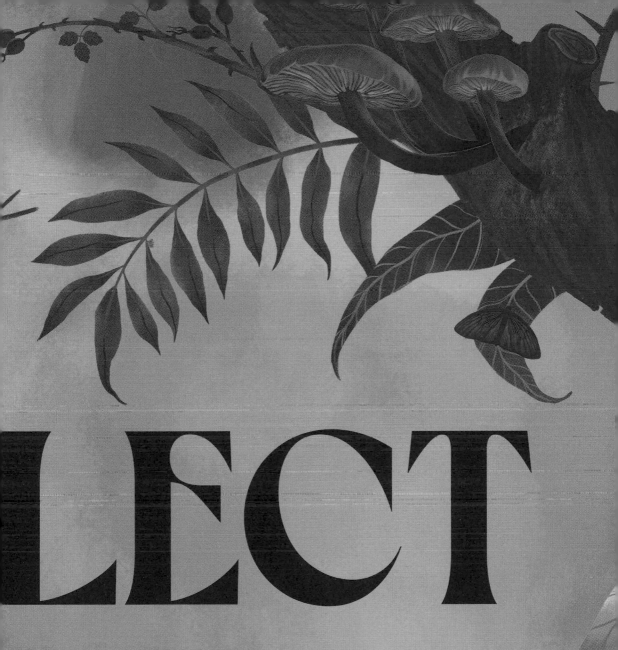

LECT

learn. The herbana witch sits by the kitchen window in the brightest spot and embroiders a butterfly on a pocket or melts wax for a balm, or even tries a new recipe. It is important to recognize one's needs and have a map of what one desires. Let it be a slow and careful harvest full of kindness, gentleness, and wonder. Move at a relaxed pace and remember that you can harvest in different ways: through photographs, drawings, notes, lists, and memories.

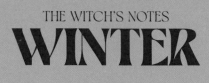

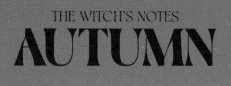

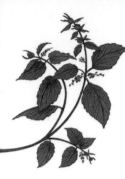

BIBLIOGRAPHY

BERNARDI, MILENA
La voce remota. La fiaba, l'infanzia, l'eredità delle storie
edizioni ETS, Pisa 2019

BOLAND, MAUREEN — BOLAND, BRIDGET
Old Wives' Lore for Gardeners
Michael O'Mara Books, 1999

CARMANA, FEDERICA
Magici incensi
Psiche 2, Turin 2009

HOOKS, BELL — NADOTTI, MARIA
Elogio del margine. Scrivere al buio
Tamu, Naples 2020

MABEY, RICHARD
Weeds: In Defense of Nature's Most Unloved Plants
Ecco, 2012

MATARRESE, ELEONORA
La cuoca selvatica. Storie e ricette per portare la natura a tavola
Bompiani, Milan 2018

MECOZZI, KARIN
Ars herbaria. Piante medicinali nel respiro dell'anno
Natura e Cultura Editrice, Alassio 2020

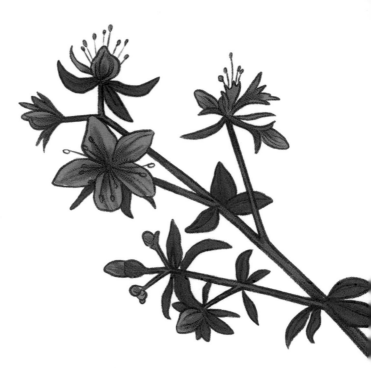

MONTGOMERY, LUCY MAUD
I boschi e le stagioni
Lindau edizioni, Turin 2022

ROBERTSON, LEEZA
Animal Totem Tarot
Llewellyn, Woodbury (Minnesota) 2016

SCOTT, DEVON
I giardini incantati le piante e la magia lunare
Venexia, Rome 2006

SIGNORINI, CARLO
Le erbe filosofia e pratica
Edizioni del Baldo, Verona 2018

STAFFORD, FIONA
The Long, Long Life of Trees
Yale University Press, 2017

VACCHETTO, MARIA IOLE
Elogio del margine. Altri modi di pensare la malattia
Associazione Primalpe Costanzo Martini, Cuneo 2016